CW01261464

The Breath of Consolation

The Breath of Consolation

Finding Solace in Cancer Literature

Josephine Brady

Josephine Brady

With a foreword by Brian Keenan

Copyright in the compilation and essays
© Josephine Brady, 2024

The moral right of Josephine Brady to be identified as the author of the essays
and compiler of this work has been asserted in accordance with
the Copyright, Designs and Patents Act of 1988.

The moral right of Brian Keenan to be identified as the author of the foreword has been asserted in
accordance with the Copyright, Designs and Patents Act of 1988.

The moral right of the contributing authors of poems and excerpts featured
in this hybrid work to be identified as such is asserted in accordance with the Copyright,
Designs and Patents Act of 1988. The list of individual titles and respective
copyrights on page 331 constitutes an extension of this copyright page.

All rights reserved. No part of this publication may be reproduced,
stored in a retrieval system, or transmitted in any form or by any means,
electronic, mechanical, photocopying, recording, or otherwise, without the prior
written permission of the copyright owner and publisher of this book.

All poems and excerpts have been reproduced according to the styles found in the original works.
As a result, some spellings and accents used can vary throughout this hybrid work.

ISBN: 978-1-3999-8518-5

Book Design by Anú Design, Tara, Ireland
Author photo by Lorraine O'Sullivan Photography
Printed and bound by L&C Printing Group, Poland

To benefit:
Cuan Cancer Support Centre, Cavan
Gary Kelly Cancer Support Centre, Drogheda

For

Paul and Kate

and all who suffer because of cancer.

Contents

Foreword by Brian Keenan   xi
Author's Note   xv

Part One: Memoirs   1

Skybound: A Journey in Flight	*Rebecca Loncraine*	7
Quicksand	*Henning Mankell*	13
Autobiography of a face	*Lucy Grealy*	17
The Audre Lorde Compendium	*Audre Lorde*	21
C: Because cowards get cancer too...	*John Diamond*	27
The Museum of Words	*Georgia Blain*	31
In your face	*Lia Mills*	37
Mortality	*Christopher Hitchens*	43
My Bright Abyss	*Christian Wiman*	47
Memoir	*John McGahern*	53

Part Two: Novels   59

The Blood of the Lamb	*Peter De Vries*	63
Between a Wolf and a Dog	*Georgia Blain*	67
Age of Iron	*J. M. Coetzee*	71
The Christmas Tree	*Jennifer Johnston*	75
A Monster Calls	*Patrick Ness*	79
The spare room	*Helen Garner*	83
The Sickness	*Alberto Barrera Tyszka*	87
So Much For That	*Lionel Shriver*	91
Gain	*Richard Powers*	95
As You Were	*Elaine Feeney*	99

Part Three: Poetry — 105

Sentenced to Life: Poems 2011–2014	*Clive James*	111
Inside the Wave *from* Counting Backwards	*Helen Dunmore*	115
The Bridge	*Marin Sorescu*	121
Say Yes Quickly: A Cancer Tapestry	*Mary Bradish O'Connor*	129
Without. Poems	*Donald Hall*	141
Of Mutability	*Jo Shapcott*	151
Every riven thing	*Christian Wiman*	159
Still Life	*Ciaran Carson*	169
First Light: A selection of poems	*Philip Hodgins*	189
All of Us: The Collected Poems	*Raymond Carver*	201

Part Four: Short Stories and Novellas — 209

A Manual for Cleaning Women: selected stories	*Lucia Berlin*	215
Grief	*Lucia Berlin*	217
Fool to Cry	*Lucia Berlin*	221
Panteón de Dolores	*Lucia Berlin*	225
Mama	*Lucia Berlin*	227
Wait a Minute	*Lucia Berlin*	229
People Like That Are the Only People Here	*Lorrie Moore*	233
I Want to Live!	*Thom Jones*	239
Floating Bridge	*Alice Munro*	243
Light	*Elizabeth Strout*	249
Tell Me a Riddle	*Tillie Olsen*	253
Muriel Scaife	*Pat Barker*	259
The Last Summer	*Bernhard Schlink*	265
Little Disturbances	*Mary Costello*	271
The Death of Ivan Ilyich	*Leo Tolstoy*	277

Part Five: Fabulous Endings — 283

The Emperor of All Maladies	*Siddhartha Mukherjee*	287
The Truth in Small Doses	*Clifton Leaf*	295
The Immortal Life of Henrietta Lacks	*Rebecca Skloot*	301
Reading and Writing Cancer	*Susan Gubar*	309
A Grief Observed	*C. S. Lewis*	315
Gratitude	*Oliver Sacks*	321

Acknowledgements — 329
Extended Copyright — 331

Foreword

Brian Keenan

Some years ago, I turned on the radio and listened in on an interview with someone called John Moriarty. I did not know who the man was as I had tuned in after the interview had started and missed the introduction. I was listening mainly because Mr Moriarty had a way of saying things that I found intriguing. However, when he started talking about his own diagnosis of cancer and how he related to it as a 'Celebration of the Mass of Cancer' that really got to me. I was angered at what I thought of as the man's pompous piety and I roared back at the radio, "Oh, yeah, go tell that to some young mother or father who has been told they are terminal and see how far your 'Celebration' gets you!" I stopped listening to the programme, thinking I couldn't bear much more of these priestly platitudes.

Sometime later, I discovered the work of John Moriarty and what a fine writer he was, who explored the far reaches of human consciousness and understanding in a deeply profound, eclectic and expansive way. His books seemed at first difficult to access, his ideas complex and esoteric, but as I persevered with him, I came to understand what a beautifully compassionate and illuminated mind he possessed. And he wasn't even a priest! But I was beginning to sense an understanding of his notion of the Celebration of the Mass of Cancer. I suppose, in a way, the experience of being given a cancer diagnosis is a bit like reading John Moriarty's books for the first time. They are not easy to come to terms with. His writings tend to take you out of whatever comfortable grounds of reasoning you clothe yourself in.

Cancer is like that. It is F...g Scary!, and you can't just shout at it like an inanimate radio in the hopes that it will go away. No, cancer is inside you, growing there. Usually, the immediate response is to feel enclosed and frozen as over the next few months a state of psychological paralysis starts gnawing at you. You become a king of Saint Sebastian shot through with the arrows of panic, fear, denial, anger, confusion, disbelief, sadness, self-pity, and regret. The isolation and loneliness are like a tightening vice and the emotional meltdown is merciless. The world around you goes on in its mundanely merry way, but you are no longer part of it. You are in a different space/time continuum, in the world but not part of it.

Slowly, after God alone knows how many dread-filled months of struggle, we begin to emerge out of our dark place and we might even have moments that seem in a way blessed. I liken it to being afloat in our soul boat and watching the dawn rise like a beautiful aria. But none of this is easy. There is no simple paint by numbers, step by step guide to dealing with THE diagnosis. There is no one size fits all. It is one step forward, two steps back, fall down, get up and start hauling the boulder up the hill again. You are now a member of the Society of Sisyphus! But one thing is sure. You are being re-made, re-structured, re- imagined. Acceptance is hard, because the battle is hard fought, and the devastation hard to look upon. But our soul boat is buoyant, we do not sink entirely!

Some months ago, I was discussing creative writing with a group of people with various mental health issues. I assured them that words were powerful medicine, more potent than traditional medicine because writing reveals parts of ourselves that have been waiting to be released. If we get lost in the raging storms of cancer, we can still WRITE OURSELVES HOME. Home is who you are or who you want to be. It is the safe harbour. Just as the pictures, the ornaments, the colour of our curtains, and all our household trivia define us, the new lingua franca that we are discovering as we write reveals a new found land that we see beyond the seeming catastrophe of cancer. It is life enhancing in a way that we could never have known before. That's the paradox that is at the heart of John Moriarty's Celebration of Cancer. The story has it that in the final months of John's life as his hair began falling out (he had a head of thick curls that no comb could tame) he would collect up these shedded strands of hair and lay them outside his house in some sheltered spot. Weeks after he was buried, a neighbour attested to finding several empty nests with the wiry threads of his hair woven into them! The writings in this collection are a bit like Moriarty's hair. They help us to build nests, a sheltering place, or what I prefer to call our soul boat. Each piece of work is soul food, provisioning for the journey out beyond where the Aria sings!

Author's Note

When cancer strikes, readers yearn for the redemptive and consoling company of great writers. This book introduces extraordinary writing about cancer across key literary genres. Commentary, anthology and personal reflection combine to provide a luminous pathway to fifty remarkable treasures. It is a gathering of imaginative and sheltering spaces of safe retreat that are imbued with emotional and intellectual honesty. Feast on their language and story. Feel the breath of consolation. This is writing that illuminates ways in which suffering can be endured, meaning found and hope recovered.

Finding the finest memoirs, novels, poetry, short stories and other literary work about cancer is no easy task. The sheer size and exponential growth of the cancer book world creates a huge challenge for any reader but most especially for those grappling with cancer. Help is needed to navigate swiftly and surely to writing that illuminates the complexities of the cancer experience. But how to discover that writing? Where to start? Which literary genres deliver what the reader living with cancer yearns for? Is it even possible to create a balance across genres that satisfies? As the questions multiplied in my mind, I was reminded of Neil Gaiman's metaphor for the difficulties posed by the vast world of books.

> The challenge becomes, not finding that scarce plant growing in the desert, but finding a specific plant growing in a jungle.

The idea for this book came to me shortly after I was diagnosed with chronic lymphocytic leukaemia (CLL), in May 2014. I suddenly found myself catapulted from what Susan Sontag memorably called the "kingdom of the well" into "the kingdom of the sick" and with no prospect of return. CLL is not a curable cancer. Its course is utterly unpredictable. It may smoulder for decades but can also take a sinister turn at any point. I struggled to come to terms with my new reality. Outwardly, I appeared stoical and in control. Inside, I was in turmoil. I felt oppressed, stranded in my own mind, troubled by unformed thoughts and unable to articulate my feelings. The assumption that I could control my own destiny had been shattered to smithereens. And with that, my sense of self was crumbling. I was also awash with guilt at my response to diagnosis. After all, my cancer path might be relatively minor. I did not have to face treatment immediately. Many people with CLL survive for years. Moreover, at the very moment I was diagnosed the medical world was reporting a paradigm shift in CLL care that offered more effective treatment and even the faint hope of a cure. What right had I to feel lost and adrift? And yet uncertainty and fear threatened to leach all colour and meaning out of my life. It was as if a layer of skin had been ripped off and I was left utterly exposed and vulnerable, swamped by an ever-present sense of dread. I had quite suddenly been "made foreign to myself"[1] by this discovery of a growing army of deviant cells in my blood, intent on colonisation and threatening to steal my present and my future. Instinctively I reached for the lifeline that has never failed me in times of personal turmoil.

The world of literature has always been my refuge, a place of shelter where I can break free of worries and be transported to another world, for a time at least. Distraction and escape are no little things but they are only a small part of what books gift us. Trauma can be addressed, even displaced. You come away carrying the words of the writer inside you and knowing that your private self has been fundamentally changed. Literature is capable of transforming traumatic experiences. Its redemptive potential should never be doubted. After diagnosis, I instinctively turned to literature as a safe space to go in search of insight, meaning and perspective. I needed words for what I was going through and wisdom that would enable me to come to terms with it. I hungered for the work of writers who understood that reconciliation with fate and recovery of hope demand fiercely honest portrayals of cancer's brutal realities. Instinctively I was drawn to writing that originated in difficult personal cancer experiences. I longed for consolation from those who have grappled with cancer and its attendant uncertainties and fears. I yearned for support in finding a pathway to recover my faith in life. I craved language that fit the intensity of what I was experiencing. Suffering is so often the inspiration for great writing. Edna O'Brien's description

---

[1] An exemplary description of the distressing impact of illness on the psyche from Hilary Mantel's memoir *Giving Up the Ghost*.

of profound writing as coming out of the "gouged times, when the heart is cut open" should also be applied to the act of reading. When the anguished writer and reader meet, the sense of joyous connection, of kinship, of no longer being alone in a dark place, is truly comforting. It is a special moment when a book takes hold of you. Suddenly, you see more clearly and your thoughts about what matters in life and death profoundly shift. It is as if this writer was waiting to speak just with you. It feels like you are in cahoots, forging meaning together. Moreover, there is no more powerful antidote for the cancer patient suffering the unrelenting onslaught of militaristic and medical language and the psychobabble of alternative healing than the rich language of literature.

Consequently, my personal quest for great cancer writing began. I longed to be told in no uncertain terms that these are the writers and works that I should read, and why. In the early weeks I was shocked at my failure to uncover a useful introductory guide to great cancer literature across key genres. This in turn triggered a memory of my fruitless search in 2008 for writing that might console the dying Irish writer Nuala O'Faolain. A personal quest quite organically morphed into the concept for a book that would bring the consoling and redemptive power of great cancer literature to every reader struggling with cancer – whether patient, carer, parent, partner, or friend. Toni Morrison's observation sprang to mind.

> If you find a book you really want to read but it hasn't been written yet, then you must write it.
>
> (*Cincinnati Enquirer*, 27th Sept 1981)

Living and dying with cancer is a lonely business. Readers should be able to swiftly access the finest literary companions. I had no illusions about the scale of the task ahead and wasn't fazed by the vast ocean that I was about to dive into. After all, I was wielding a public librarian's formidable arsenal for bringing people and literature together. I found purpose and focus in cutting through the noise and marketing ploys and overcoming the tyranny of the contemporary. Uncovering long-forgotten and out-of-print literary gems and slowly putting structure on the chaos of the cancer book world was deeply satisfying. Cancer had abruptly ended my career as a librarian but my drive to bring readers and remarkable books together remains as strong as ever. The urge to connect with readers is such an instinctive and passionate part of me now that it will not be ignored. I felt driven to do what I've been doing all my professional life, namely, shining a spotlight on brilliant writing. I embraced the challenge and brought every ounce of passion, integrity and commitment that I possess into play. I never imagined, however, that this quest would turn into an odyssey, albeit one interrupted in fits and starts by cancer treatment. What's more, it is an odyssey that shows no signs of ending. This book no longer feels like the final destination I expected to reach. Rather, it has turned out to be a resting place. The journey through cancer literature continues.

The intensity of my engagement with cancer literature made it the richest and most satisfying time of my reading life. A powerful literary lifeline of cancer literature slowly revealed itself. It is a lifeline that stretches back in time and reaches across borders and genres. The echoes of earlier work can be clearly heard in the words of later writers who have absorbed what past masters have to say. I found no easy comfort or trite answers to the existential questions that cancer raises. What I did encounter was writing that reminds us of humanity's shared fragility and sheds light on the mysteries of serious illness and mortality. I read everything I could, as deeply as I could. It has fundamentally altered my way of thinking about myself and our precarious and unpredictable world. This may sound overblown, I guess. Yet, cancer literature is the constant companion that has never failed me since diagnosis. It is difficult to explain quite how extraordinary cancer writing pours into the reader's soul. Although details may dim, something precious lingers and takes root. I found language and story that liberated me, providing an invaluable means of understanding myself. I've been brought home in the truest sense of the word - I am stronger, calmer and better prepared for whatever life brings. When darkness gathers, cancer writing invariably steers me out of a fog of despair and towards the light. It prompts me to accept uncertainty. In consequence, co-existing with painful realities has become easier. I am reminded that resolution may not always be possible and everything in life is fundamentally groundless in any case. It nudges me to live in the present moment and focus on the goodness and richness that remains in my life. My reading odyssey nourishes and nurtures me, effectively rescuing me from trauma time and again. It truly is soul medicine that never fails to heal. So, I am determined to share a select company of writers that I have come to love with you. I know that it will help you navigate through the cancer abyss, replenish your spirit, and create the inner resources desperately needed in order to recover hope and endure. You will emerge with a better understanding of life, of mortality and of yourself.

This book rests heavily on the shoulders of all the writers I encountered who made it nigh on impossible to limit my selection to just fifty great reads. The final works are a seriously considered sample of literary gold, drawn from the broadest spectrum of cancer writing from across the world and through time. Cancer literature from three centuries, six continents, thirteen countries and key genres feature. Classics of the cancer canon together with landmark works that critiqued cancer culture are given prominence. World-renowned writers are intermingled with authors largely unknown beyond national borders or academic circles. Fresh new voices are juxtaposed with writers of towering presence whose books are the crowning achievements of distinguished writing careers. A deeply satisfying feature is the inclusion of neglected novelists, poets, memoirists and journalists whose writing is arresting and accomplished. Marginalised voices speak loudly. I am pleased but not at all surprised that six Irish writers feature and that a scrupulously gender-blind selection process resulted in a near-perfect balance.

As diverse as the writers who created them, all fifty works nevertheless share certain invaluable qualities. All deal unflinchingly with the pain and suffering of cancer and break the culture of silence around death. Critical concerns are teased out and placed centre stage. Cancer's difficult, often frightening and sometimes disfiguring physical impacts are powerfully conveyed. Writers struggling with existential crises bring clarity and insight to spiritual and philosophical questions. The emotional challenges cancer imposes on friendships and family relationships are astutely explored. Thorny issues such as the tyranny of positivity, quack medicine, the battlefield language of cancer and the role of patient advocacy are all addressed. The chosen writers do not simplify the cancer experience. Rather, they broaden it out, embracing its complexity and distilling hard-won wisdom. A wonderful sense of solidarity is tangible. This is writing that answers our aching need for some kind of immutable consolation. A permanent resource that we can return to time and again, it speaks to our souls and we feel the breath of consolation.

Although darkness, fear and dread are present, reading these works is as far from bleak as you can possibly imagine. This company of writers cuts through personal loneliness and despair and enables the reader to "see into the life of things", as Wordsworth so beautifully expressed it. Wit, black humour, honesty and quirkiness abound. Paradoxically, in looking suffering and death in the face it is also life that is examined and celebrated. It is profoundly reassuring to find that we are in fact reading love letters to life and all that makes it so richly meaningful. Who would have thought that great cancer writing could be suffused with gratitude, and yes, even joy?

However pleasurable and inspiring research and reading proved to be, the writing process was an altogether different story. Although I never once lost faith in the book's concept, nor in the writing selected, I had doubts about my ability to do justice to both. Still, the instinctive feel for what readers love, honed over a career as a public librarian and a lifetime as a devoted reader, would not be discounted. What kept me going was my conviction that ordinary readers desperately need this resource. I am no academic. I'm simply another ordinary reader, as so perfectly described by Colm Tóibín in *A Guest at the Feast*.

> She was what most writers long for, and what most of us still write for: the ordinary reader, curious and intelligent and demanding, ready to be moved and changed, and believing still that the written word has all the power to make the deepest imprint on the private self.

The final result is a gathering of literary voices that is a sturdy bridge to cancer literature's long-established lifeline. Writers with vastly different cancer perspectives speak directly to our souls, imparting wisdom and solace. Drawing inspiration from Helen Dunmore, I see the selected writers as custodians of the space between light and darkness and every work as a stepping-stone that illuminates the way.

I began with the lofty ambition of producing a definitive introductory collection – the last word, if you will – on cancer literature. I soon realised that this was a foolhardy mission. My compilation is simply a starting point, a subjective choice mirroring the person I am and the experiences that have shaped me. This individual quality is both the book's strength and its weakness. I know that readers adore lists, reading guides and anthologies. Helping readers navigate through the labyrinthine book world to great writing is their compilers' shared ambition. Preventing readers from losing sight of works that matter is a key aim. Selected works are usually hotly debated and sometimes controversial. Noting absences and disagreeing with choices is simply part of the fun. My hope is that this book too will generate such criticism. Even better, it may lead others to create new bridges to great cancer literature for readers to delight in. After all, those of us living and dying with cancer will be the ultimate beneficiaries.

An ancient Egyptian library had the words "The Place of the Cure of the Soul" inscribed on its entrance. It is a fitting description of what librarians down through history have aspired to create. Those words also perfectly capture what I set out to achieve for cancer literature with this book. When we feel imprisoned by despair and cut off from the world, the alchemy of great cancer writing unfetters us. It heals our despair. It restores the possibility of becoming, as was so perfectly expressed by Emily Brontë, "chainless souls", with the strength to endure whatever cancer may have in store.

PART 1

Memoirs

Introduction

It seemed simple at first. My aim was clear. Find brilliant cancer memoirs that have the capacity to change how the reader sees and understands their own cancer experience and, in so doing, help the reader to find solace in the midst of suffering. What was hazy, however, was exactly how to achieve it. Although I had some inkling of the scale of the task, I was quickly overwhelmed by a tsunami of memoirs that continued to grow over my ten-year reading odyssey. Even well-honed librarian skills proved unequal to the task.

I started by identifying the themes and perspectives that commonly appear in cancer memoirs. The story that frequently unfolds is of the journey from symptoms to diagnosis and treatment, and on to recovery or decline. Anger at and scepticism about the medical establishment together with the urgent need for self-advocacy regularly feature and often make for riveting reading. The thorny subjects of assisted suicide and euthanasia have been explored. Unsurprisingly, the financial catastrophe wrought by cancer is a feature of many American memoirs but it also has a presence in some European memoirs. The perspectives of both cancer patients and cancer carers can be found in even the earliest published accounts. Gender-specific, age-specific and cancer-specific memoirs have proliferated. Memoirs have been written by people from all walks of life, including celebrities. The insider perspective provided by the doctor-turned-patient has an understandable attraction for readers. Members of ethnic and racial groups who are disproportionately impacted by cancer as a result of discrimination have written movingly about their experiences.

I am convinced that there is merit to be found in nearly all published memoirs and the creation of such work is, at the very minimum, empowering for the writer. Every memoirist has their unique experience to share. Readers yearn to enter and explore another human being's experience of cancer. As someone who could never bleed on the page, unable to write about my personal cancer experience, I am in awe of the raw courage of so many memoirists. The key question is how to represent not only the diversity but also the commonality of themes and perspectives in just ten memoirs. Selection criteria had to be found to ensure well-directed and productive research. Both positive and negative principles emerged in response to this quandary.

The list of 'negative' principles developed and applied was relatively short. Quickly dismissed were all memoirs that had even a whiff of a happy-clappy, 'positive thinking' vibe or used the battle language of cancer. Readers daily encounter more than enough of the "you can beat it – stay positive" language. The tyranny of cheerfulness is a feature of many cancer memoirs and can be truly damaging. Its presence meant immediate elimination. Pedestrian writing offering little or no perspective and adding nothing of perceptible value, together with works suffused with self-pity or sickly-sweet sentiment, were rejected. Memoirs that embrace alternative medicine and the anti-medical dogma so dangerous for cancer patients had no place. All of this helped reduce the mountain of material under consideration. Three 'positive' principles were then brought into play to ensure that only the finest material would be considered. Ten years on, I am quietly confident that these positive principles were a saving grace and broke the necessary ground, creating a clear pathway to the final selection.

So, what were these positive principles? The overriding one was that the memoir's author had to have a great writing style. Readers who love literature both need and want a cancer experience to be expressed by a skilled and creative wordsmith. Expertly chosen words and phrases used within a well thought out narrative structure are always a joy to read. The art of expressing experience matters and is no little thing. That art brings with it the power to make the reader live, feel and enter fully into the writer's experience. When I finally reached the shortlist stage, I found that, without consciously pre-determining it, every title selected was the work of a poet, a novelist or a journalist. I shouldn't have been surprised. After all, the ability to imbue language with meaning is the writer's art.

Tied to writing style was the second principle: the skill of making sense of a personal cancer experience in terms of larger truths. Cancer and its treatment result in unwanted, difficult, often frightening and sometimes disfiguring physical changes. The corrosive psychological and emotional scars are much harder to pin down and probe, however. We look to creative minds to help us grapple with the myriad of issues that bubble beneath the surface reality of physical pain and suffering. Readers need support in coping with the loss of a sense of self; living with fear, uncertainty and vulnerability; and coming to terms with mortality. Great cancer memoir writing does not simplify the cancer experience but broadens it out, embracing its complexity. From that complexity, philosophical considerations of living and dying with cancer are distilled into hard-won wisdom. This can be profoundly empowering. The reader sees more clearly and reaches a better understanding of themselves and their own responses to cancer.

The third principle was that four key sub-genres – pioneering memoirs; gender-specific memoirs; memoirs focused on spirituality; memoirs by journalists – all had to feature. The historically and culturally important landmark works that critiqued cancer culture, and in so doing, effectively changed the field of cancer literature forever, had to be represented. So too the large sub-genre written exclusively by women that focus on gender-specific cancers. Reconnecting with our spiritual selves is a matter of deep concern for many, so memoirs exploring spirituality, belief and unbelief were essential. Finally, the sub-genre of memoirs produced by journalists are distinct in style and substance from the work of other writers and merited inclusion. I must admit that I have a weakness for great journalism, married as I am to a dedicated and skilful journalist! Many of the common themes and perspectives mentioned previously were addressed in the memoirs selected to represent these pivotal sub-genres.

A shortlist of over thirty titles gradually took shape. The Memoirs section proved by far the most challenging to whittle down. Rejecting so many exceptional memoirs was difficult and there is no doubt that excellence exists well beyond the titles chosen. However, the final ten are the memoirs that I loved most and felt absolutely compelled to persuade others to read. I returned to them time and again, always finding something fresh in these intensely human accounts of the bleakest of human experiences.

Skybound: A Journey in Flight (2018)

Rebecca Loncraine

(*British writer 1974–2016*)

Choosing the two works to bookend this section required serious thought. All of the memoirs featured are exceptional and any one of the ten could easily sit in either spot. It seemed that this conundrum was impossible to solve, a little like picking a favourite child. There is an entirely appropriate poignancy to the rationale arrived at to resolve the issue. The author chosen to feature first was at the start of a promising writing career, with just one work published, when she was diagnosed with breast cancer. Her second book, *Skybound*, was published posthumously and is, quite simply, a glorious act of healing. Loncraine was a hugely talented author whose writing potential was lost to the world just as her career was taking off. The author who features last is, by contrast, a towering presence in English literature. His memoir is the crowning achievement of a career in which his writing promise was fully realised. And yet, both memoirs share important qualities. In writing about the devastating impact of cancer on their lives, the two writers evoke a love of place, a spiritual connectedness to the landscape of home, and a deep appreciation for the natural world. There is also a quiet joy and a sense of calm acceptance, born out of suffering, that make both works deeply consoling reads.

Rebecca Loncraine worked hard to establish a writing career. After attending art school, she studied History and English, and achieved a doctorate in English literature. A career as a freelance writer followed. Supported by grant aid, she researched and published her first work, a literary biography of L. Frank Baum (creator of *The Wizard of Oz*) and was working on further projects while living with her partner in Oxford. A breast cancer diagnosis in 2009 blew everything apart. The life plan disintegrated and she moved back to her family farm in Wales for a gruelling year of chemotherapy, surgery, and radiotherapy. Traumatised by cancer and rendered almost speechless by the horrors of treatment, the desire to write seemed to have deserted her.

> I was discovering that disease may manifest in the body, but it's a profoundly psychological, emotionally charged experience, that shakes you right down to the bedrock.

Returning to her old life was all but impossible as she struggled to find a way back to living fully, with no idea how to even start. That is until April 2011, when, while out walking with friends, she passed the Black Mountains Gliding Club. The decision to fly was born out of her desperate need to find some way to rise above the grief of her cancer experience. Her first flight proved unforgettable and left her euphoric.

> My relationship with fear and risk had totally altered: cancer had stripped away any delusion of safety on the ground. Suddenly, I wanted to face fear head on – to choose it, move towards it, become intimate with it – and, in this choosing, I hoped I might find some freedom from it.

Loncraine's endeavour to learn to fly proved transformative. Slowly released from the grip of grief and fear, she re-engaged with the natural world and found a way to accept her mortality, yet still live joyously. The language she had been searching for to speak about trauma emerged and, with it, the desire to write.

> ... flying is helping me come to terms with the changes the illness has wrought in me physically and psychologically ... I start talking about my own experience, about the fear and loneliness of cancer, about the shame of it and the sheer exhausting drudgery of treatment.

A creative defence against the battle language surrounding cancer is ably mounted in the book.

> After the diagnosis, many kind and supportive people told me I was in a 'battle' with cancer, and would advise me about the skills needed to 'fight' the disease. It was a language of violence and conquest. I was encouraged to 'know my enemy'. I took quite the opposite approach: surrender, gentleness and vulnerability. In not fighting, I found a quiet attentiveness to the present moment and an intense intimacy with the world that revealed a raw toughness at my core, which gave me enormous strength to endure.

Skybound is so much more than a memoir of illness and many subjects are capably interwoven into its structure. Loncraine is, at different moments, a naturist, a travel writer, a botanist, a geographer, a learner aviator, and a historian exploring the history of unpowered flight. Perspectives on her cancer experience are interwoven into the fabric of the narrative.

> Flying brings you into greater intimacy with nature. That's what I've been searching for, up here. The natural world can hold any hurt inside it, recognise it, gently turn it over in the palm of its hand like a precious stone, and I have the sense now that the sky has crept up into my spine, worked its blue way into my bones.

It is the mark of a great storyteller when a reader becomes enraptured by a world previously taken for granted and poorly understood. Loncraine is awed by the nature of the sky and the allure of unpowered flight. As she navigates the sky, she captures our imagination with astonishing descriptive passages. We learn about ridge air, thermal lift, convergence lift, cloud formations, and what all of this means for the flyer. Illness has altered her sense of time and she responds with joy on finding that in the air time becomes elastic and utterly different from time as experienced on the ground.

Travel writing at its finest emerges as Loncraine's experience of unpowered flight unfolds. Her account of gliding in Wales, New Zealand and Nepal is exquisitely told. Unadulterated pleasure awaits the reader as Loncraine interacts with the sheer beauty of the world as seen from the unique perspective of the sky. She brings us right into her cockpit on a tour of the skies and the ever-changing landscapes of the earth below. We soar with her over not only the Black Mountains of Wales but also the dramatic locations of New Zealand's Southern Alps and the Nepalese Himalayas. The shapes of rivers and lakes;

the peaks of mountain ranges; the varieties of plant life and their abundance of colour appear vividly in our imagination, placed there by Loncraine's poetic prose. Fresh and interesting perspectives on the earth below her are powerfully portrayed, tangled up with childhood memories and cancer experiences.

> I'm shocked to suddenly notice that we're flying directly over my home ∴.. I trace the boundaries of the farm with my finger from inside the glider. I see how the land rises up and wraps around it on three sides, so it looks like it's held in the cupped hand of the hill. Beyond the form, I can see how it sits within the landscape, and I've a feeling of rediscovering my familiar world, but from a much larger perspective.

She juxtaposes the damage wrought by radiation with the devastation of hill fires.

> The more I look at it, the more the scar on the hill and my own scar start to feel like openings for painful truths to enter. Illness is part of nature, as are hill fires.

Particularly touching are the passages about Loncraine's encounters with birdlife, both on the ground and in the air. Months of treatment result in a growing appreciation for garden birds including starlings, robins and wrens and also for the wonderful dawn chorus. In the air, she flies alongside the red kites of Wales; and abroad, shares the sky with griffon vultures and buzzards. Pure magic emanates from her description of feeding a rescue vulture from a paraglider in Nepal.

> He lands perfectly on my hand, decelerating from seventy kilometres an hour in a matter of seconds. He snatches the meat and then swoops off the gloved hand to the left and is swallowed again in the sky's currents, which have become as thick as water at this speed.

Through scholarly research she presents the reader with quirky stories of historical figures enamoured with flying. We are also left in no doubt about the present-day dangers extreme flyers are exposed to in the most daunting flying locations in the world.

Loncraine is transformed by the experience of unpowered flight and its consequential impact on her sense of self. *Skybound* is also a profound love letter to the natural world and life in all its forms. The rediscovery of personal joy is uplifting. The dignified acceptance of uncertainty and frailty as a natural part of living and dying is something readers living with cancer will admire and also aspire to. As Loncraine was finishing this memoir, cancer returned. She underwent a further fourteen months of treatment but died at home in Wales in September 2016, aged just forty-two. *Skybound* has a freshness and beauty rarely seen so early in a writer's career. At its very heart, the inner journey of self-discovery is inextricably bound up with the odyssey into the sky and the world of unpowered flight. Loncraine excels in the telling of both tales. The result is a beautifully written cancer memoir which is unique, wise, joyous, and utterly unforgettable.

Quicksand: What it Means to Be a Human Being (2014)

Henning Mankell
(*Swedish writer 1948–2015*)

Laurie Thompson
(*British translator 1938–2015*)

It is rare to find a cancer memoir that breaks free from the well-trodden chronological path of diagnosis, treatment, untold suffering and eventual recovery or decline. The remarkable sixty-seven essays of *Quicksand* are a world away from that model. Mankell chooses instead to bring the reader on a reflective journey that moves seamlessly through time, history and place. As he delves into memories of a rich and fulfilling life, we are transported across Europe and to East Africa and encounter both the creativity and the destructiveness that human beings have wrought on earth. From cave paintings and the treasures of the Louvre and the Prado, to nuclear waste storage in Finnish mountain tunnels and human catastrophes, the joy and suffering Mankell has seen and experienced is laid bare. We are with Mankell as he takes his meditative journey, weighing up what he has learned about humanity and its place in planet earth's evolving story. Present throughout is a consciousness of the significance of one man's life, however transient it may be, and of the responsibility we all bear for each other and for those yet to come. Even as he writes through a cancer experience that he feels has already set him apart, he is eager for connection and engagement. Mankell shares his thoughts and feelings as death approaches with clarity and candour. As he draws from his abundant well of memories, he shows an intensity of awareness that is deeply moving. By the book's end it is as if we are reluctantly bidding farewell to an erudite, eloquent, moral and serious companion whose company has enriched our lives.

Known to many readers for his Inspector Wallander series of bestselling books, Henning Mankell was diagnosed with incurable lung cancer in 2013, underwent treatment, but died in the Autumn of 2015. A prolific writer, Mankell was also a human rights activist, deeply concerned about the inequalities in this world and determined to do what he could to bring about real change. Using the fortune generated from his writing, he endowed an orphanage in Mozambique, funded the arts in Sweden and in Africa, and established and managed a theatre, also in Mozambique. Actively involved in left-wing politics from his youth, he campaigned for many causes including raising awareness of the Aids epidemic and the landmines crisis. He was committed to the Palestinian cause and in 2010 took part in the Gaza Freedom Flotilla. In short, he was a remarkable man, living a fully engaged life. Until, that is, he received a cancer diagnosis. In searching for words to express his feelings on diagnosis, he found the title for this memoir.

> What I felt was precisely that fear of quicksand. I fought against being sucked down and swallowed up by it. By the totally paralysing realisation that I had been stricken by a serious, incurable disease. It took me ten days and nights, with very few hours of sleep, to keep myself afloat and not be incapacitated by the fear that threatened to overcome all my powers of resistance ... In the end I was able to crawl back out of the sand and begin to come to terms with what had happened.

Not surprisingly, for a man whose life demonstrated a determination to face difficulties and injustices head on, he found the strength to continue to do so when faced with cancer. It is moving to read how he handled the paralysing panic and fear many readers are so familiar with. He did so with a razor-sharp focus on living an ethical life.

> I started to formulate questions about courage and fear ... Courage and fear are always intertwined. It requires courage to live and courage

to die ... No doubt I am afraid. High storm waves could come from nowhere at any moment and crash against my inner and outer coastlines ... If the worst should happen, if the cancerous tumours multiply and can't be stopped, I shall die. There is nothing I can do, apart from summoning up the courage that is necessary to lead a decent life. Sometimes, especially during the night, I wake up in a state of almost panic-stricken worry. It usually doesn't take long for me to become calm again – a fragile calm, but calm even so.

As Mankell writes about living and dying with cancer, he does so honestly and unflinchingly but without a scintilla of self-pity. Readers living with cancer will recognise the commonality of many experiences. In writing about what cancer reveals about our relationships he does not shy away from exposing his personal hurt and disappointment.

Some reacted as one would expect: with sympathy, worry and friendly understanding. Others simply disappeared. Ceased to get in touch ... I admit that I have been surprised in recent times. People I thought might flee into the shadows have proved to be strong enough to remain in touch, while others of whom I expected more have disappeared over the horizon ... But I don't pass judgement on anybody. People are who they are. One doesn't need to have many friends – but one should be able to rely on those one has ...

Mankell is convinced that books and storytelling are essential to life and are powerful tools in countering the harrowing realities of living and dying with cancer. He recounts how buying books before a cycle of chemotherapy not only comforted him but also acted as an advance reward for what he was about to go through. The joy Mankell finds in re-reading much loved novels such as Robinson Crusoe is also touchingly conveyed.

I am constantly reminded that we human beings are basically storytellers. More *Homo narrans* than *Homo sapiens*. We see ourselves in others' stories ... With books it was possible to counter the almost intolerable pressure to devote all my attention to the disease, the treatment, and constantly looking for signs of new symptoms ... I was not simply a person who had been diagnosed with a serious illness: I was also the same person as I had been before, myself and no other. It was possible to live in two worlds at the same time.

As Mankell casts an impassioned eye on life and death, he finds a perspective that is both unambiguous and deeply consoling. The human lifespan is very short and insignificant in and of itself. It should be seen in the wider context of the continuity of the human story, linked as we all are to the generations before and after our own brief timeframe on this earth. Seeing a single life from this viewpoint, Mankell argues that concern should turn outward and away from ourselves to those suffering injustices and indifference, and to the environment upon which our world relies. Aware of what a privilege it is to be able to consider the meaning of life, he reminds us that millions have no such right, instead spending their whole lifetime in a fight for survival.

There is a strong sense throughout of a man condensing the hard-won wisdom of a lifetime into words, to bring clarity not only for himself as he faces the reality of approaching death, but for his readers. The essence of this singular, contemplative and talented writer is beautifully revealed. When he seeks to pinpoint the happiest moment of his life, his choice is at once unsurprising and uplifting. His encounter with pure joy is so touching that it will not be revealed in these pages. Rather, I would entreat readers to find it for themselves where it properly awaits them, in the pages of *Quicksand*.

Autobiography of a Face (1994)

Lucy Grealy

(Irish American writer 1963–2002)

Finding Lucy Grealy's memoir was a singular moment of discovery on my ten-year journey through cancer literature. It is always wise to sit up and take notice when a memoir is written by a poet and *Autobiography of a Face* not only lives up to expectations but exceeds them. It is an exquisitely written sequence of essays by a talented Irish American poet and essayist. Grealy explores her childhood and young adult years, blighted as they were by a rare cancer diagnosis, brutal treatments, facial disfigurement and many largely fruitless reconstructive surgeries. In a world obsessed with physical beauty, she reflects on the nightmare of looking physically different and the subsequent struggle to establish and accept her own identity. Feeling ugly and different brought such intense suffering that it overshadowed even the darkest moments of cancer treatment. It was not cancer that she saw as the great tragedy of her life but the reality of living with disfigurement. Dark and disturbing subject matter it may be, but somehow Grealy transforms it into content that engages and enthrals the reader in equal measure. Her voice is crystal clear, honed through prolonged bitter experiences and also through a writing talent nurtured by study and an expansive reading life. Quirky, witty, fiercely intelligent and alive to the joys of life, this unique perspective on childhood cancer and its lifelong ramifications is a standout in the world of cancer literature.

Grealy throws us into the heart of her personal tragedy from the very first essay. Finding solace in the company of animals, she worked during her childhood years at pony parties, learning early on what disfigurement does to human interactions. Enabling readers to quickly identify with her, Grealy then brings us back to what led to disfigurement. Born in Dublin in 1963, Grealy moved with her family to America when she was four. Aged just nine, she was diagnosed with the rare cancer Ewing sarcoma. In the early 1970s, treatment for Ewing sarcoma was primitive and Grealy's experiences of radical surgery, radiation and chemotherapy were at the extreme end of the spectrum. Compounding the physical horror was the emotional trauma caused by a woeful lack of understanding about the special needs of children dealing with cancer. It is to some degree understandable but nonetheless distressing to read of the multiple ways in which her parents and doctors failed her. Grealy's memories of her first hospital visit for radical surgery to remove a substantial part of her right jawbone illustrate the abject failure to properly prepare her for what lay ahead. From the present-day perspective, it is difficult to countenance. When her parents leave her on her own in the hospital, she is panic-stricken. At diagnosis, this nine-year-old is informed by her doctor that she has a malignancy. No one uses the word cancer. No attempt is made to explain what lies ahead. This bright child is not encouraged to ask questions but is instead left in a fog of misunderstanding. Many months later Grealy hears the word cancer used for the first time in reference to herself and is stunned. Her family is incredulous that she did not know.

As Grealy starts chemotherapy, yet again totally unprepared, her distraught mother unwittingly causes further significant harm, telling her daughter to deal with her fears by suppressing the urge to cry. It is a salutary reminder of the power of language for anyone caring for a child going through cancer treatment. It is a testament to her innate courage and stoicism – and perhaps also to the optimism of youth – that she managed to endure these years of great physical pain and suffering. Her reflections on the harsh reality of her treatments are astute and utterly convincing. Grealy also turns away from self-pity, not one note of which can be found in this extraordinary memoir. Her sense of humour provides much-needed relief. Another tragedy unfolds, however, when Grealy finds herself trapped behind a disfigured face which she hates and for which she is viciously and mercilessly tormented at school and in public places. She finds solace in reading and later, as she revels in a newfound talent, in writing.

After years of struggle, Grealy tasted success with an article in Harper's Magazine which in turn led to a book contract and so to publication of this memoir. She relished the critical acclaim and the brief period of happiness it brought. However, years of surgeries and the titanic struggle of living with disfigurement had left her depressed and addicted to prescription drugs. Tragically, this led to heroin addiction and Grealy died from an overdose in 2002. The world lost her unique writing talent but her life force, so magnificently captured in this luminous and riveting memoir, lives on. It is breathful of life.

The Audre Lorde Compendium (1996)

Audre Lorde
(American writer 1934–1992)

Within the memoir genre there is a large sub-genre written exclusively by women that focuses on three gender-specific cancers – breast, uterine and ovarian cancer. Second-wave feminism freed women from the silence around many previously taboo subjects including cancer. Slowly at first, autobiographical narratives about these gender-specific cancers began to appear. By the 1990s that growth was exponential, facilitated by an interesting range of factors. A vibrant women's health movement with support networks and agencies; cancer treatment advances and improving survival rates; cultural interest in confessional literature; and the growth in reality television all played a role. This complex mix of circumstances ensured ready publishers and audiences. As a result, there are many moving and well-written testimonies in print. Selecting just one outstanding memoir to represent this sub-genre seemed an impossible task. Until, that is, I read a pioneering and exemplary landmark work by a gifted poet. Audre Lorde's body of work about her breast cancer experience has emotional and intellectual intensity and is imbued with honesty, vulnerability, passion and purpose. Although the treatment landscape has changed significantly since Lorde's cancer experience (1978 to 1992), the theory underpinning her work and the essence of what she has to say remain as relevant and as potent as ever.

The author of critically acclaimed and award-winning poetry and prose, Lorde rejected categorisation and always introduced herself with a long list, celebrating every aspect of herself equally. She was a poet; a librarian; an academic; a teacher; a political thinker; a human rights activist; a lesbian; a feminist; a mother; and a black woman living with cancer. Lorde's work is best considered holistically as she fused her experience of living with cancer into her identity and it served as a catalyst for much of her work. *The Audre Lorde Compendium* is made up of three previously published titles. *The Cancer Journals* (1980) contains journal entries and short essays written between 1978 and 1979 that deal with her struggle to accept and come to terms with a breast cancer diagnosis and mastectomy. *A Burst of Light* (1988) continues her writing on living with cancer following its recurrence. *Sister Outsider* (1984) provides further insights into her cancer experience through her essays and speeches.

Lorde's approach is clear from the start of the first work, *Cancer Journals*. She shared with Susan Sontag a determination to decry the silence around, and the stigmatising nature of, cancer experiences in the late 1970s. She differed from Sontag, however, in her willingness to analyse and document her own emotional struggles. True to her activist nature, she was determined to scrutinise her pain, fear and despair and find its meaning within her life. Converting that meaning into empowering knowledge, and then language, proved useful not only for herself but for others. Her writing about cancer was self-healing. It also transformed personal experience into inspiring public and political testimony.

> Each woman responds to the crisis that breast cancer brings to her life out of a whole pattern, which is the design of who she is and how her life has been lived. The weave of her everyday existence is the training ground for how she handles crisis ... I am a post-mastectomy woman who believes our feelings need voice in order to be recognised, respected, and of use. I do not wish my anger and pain and fear about cancer to fossilise into yet another silence, nor to rob me of whatever strength can lie at the core of this experience, openly acknowledged and examined.

There is no mistaking Lorde's vulnerability nor the depth of feelings she finds difficult to communicate. She expresses her experience brilliantly through haunting images and metaphors, without an ounce of self-pity.

> I handle the outward motions of each day while pain fills me like a puspocket and every touch threatens to breach the taut membrane that keeps it from flowing through and poisoning my whole existence.

> Sometimes despair sweeps across my consciousness like luna winds across a barren moonscape. Ironshod horses rage back and forth over every nerve.

She confronts fear head on and struggles to continue to live authentically.

> Sometimes fear stalks me like another malignancy, sapping energy and power and attention from my work. A cold becomes sinister; a cough, lung cancer; a bruise, leukaemia. Those fears are most powerful when they are not given voice, and close upon their heels comes the fury that I cannot shake them. I am learning to live beyond fear by living through it, and in the process learning to turn fury at my own limitations into some more creative energy … If I cannot banish fear completely, I can learn to count with it less. For then fear becomes not a tyrant against which I waste my energy fighting, but a companion, not particularly desirable, yet one whose knowledge can be useful.

Emotional honesty is sustained but with a palpably increased sense of urgency in *A Burst of Light*. In her struggles to deal with the trauma of metastasised cancer, her voice rings out, as fresh and relevant today as when she first put pen to paper.

> One of the hardest things to accept is learning to live with uncertainty and neither deny it or hide behind it … to listen to the messages of uncertainty without allowing them to immobilise me, nor keep me from the certainties of those truths in which I believe … This is my life. Every hour is a possibility not to be banked. My most deeply held convictions and beliefs can be equally expressed in how I deal with chemotherapy as well as in how I scrutinise a poem. It's about trying to know who I am wherever I am.

I relish Lorde's determination to live fully. Her words are like a call to action that rouse and mobilise not only the writer herself but also her readers.

> I want to live the rest of my life, however long or short, with as much sweetness as I can decently manage, loving all the people I love, and doing as much as I can of the work I still have to do. I am going to write fire until it comes out my ears, my eyes, my noseholes –

everywhere. Until it's every breath I breathe. I'm going to go out like a fucking meteor!

For Lorde, it was imperative to transform silence and fear into language and action. Time and again, Lorde declared that personal scrutiny and self-revelation, difficult as it was to write, was done in the context of its usefulness for others with cancer. She rejected the silence surrounding cancer and illness on behalf of all women. How important that message of breaking the silence and speaking out remains, given women's experiences right up to the present. Lorde would have applauded Vicky Phelan for her determination and courage in breaking the silence around the cervical cancer scandal in Ireland. Silence in all aspects of life remains one of the forces used against women and Lorde's critiques of dominance and exploitation retain their validity.

A self-advocate when dealing with the medical establishment long before it became fashionable to be so, she helped pave the way for women to speak up and demand a part in the decision-making process about their own bodies, their own health. She gave witness to the flaws in the systems and agencies, challenging the American Cancer Society for its failure to deal with cancer prevention and exposing Cancer Support organisations for their lack of awareness of racial, sexual and cultural differences.

Scepticism about conventional medicine and a willingness to embrace alternative treatments feature in her writing. She was determined to consider all options and make informed decisions to maximise her chances of survival.

Lorde understood the significance of difference in all its forms and fervently believed that society should not only value but also grasp the opportunities difference offers for societal growth. She rejected the cultural demand that women look a certain way, refusing a prosthesis, thereby refusing to render her difference invisible or to have her identity defined by her external appearance. Her determination to identify as one-breasted was also a gesture of solidarity with other post-mastectomy women. Lorde's refusal to allow cancer to engulf her life radiates through all three works. From the moment of diagnosis, she wrestled with the question of how her cancer experiences fitted into the larger picture of her work but also into the history of women in general. She continued to write until virtually the moment of her death.

> Living a self-conscious life, under the pressure of time, I work with the consciousness of death at my shoulder, not constantly, but often

enough to leave a mark upon all of my life's decisions and actions. And it does not matter whether this death comes next week or thirty years from now; this consciousness gives my life breadth. It helps shape the words I speak, the ways I love, my politic of action, the strength of my vision and purpose, the depth of my appreciation for living.

Lorde's poetic voice, intellectual strength, emotional intelligence and passion for life ensure that her work retains all of its force. It should find a readership for generations to come. Certainly, no woman with cancer could find a more sustaining companion in print.

C: Because cowards get cancer too ... (1998)

John Diamond

(English writer 1953–2001)

A discernible grouping within the memoir genre that deserves separate consideration is the autobiographical work of journalists living and dying with cancer. There has been an explosion of such memoirs, many of which originate in newspaper columns that at a later stage are shaped into books. Cancer memoirs by journalists have a very distinct feel and the reader is guaranteed quite a different reading experience. In the very best of such memoirs all the elements of great journalism feature. Unique writing skills are brought to bear including adept storytelling with an immediacy that hooks – and holds – the reader. The reporter's innate curiosity, analytical approach and determination to understand the disease first and then illuminate the subject with professionally researched facts, is apparent. Present also are journalistic abilities to source, to interrogate, to evaluate, to navigate and finally to effectively communicate the complex nature of living with cancer. The reporter's adoption of a personal tone when reporting on their own cancer experiences ensures that the reader is fully invested at all times. A 'warts and all' approach gives a sense of intimate connection. With memoirs that start life as newspaper columns, interaction often takes place between the journalist and readers who regularly respond to the columns by email and letter. These responses influence the writing of subsequent columns and so in turn subtly shape the final book. In many such memoirs there is a real sense of a conversation taking place, of one human being who can write well speaking directly and intimately with the reader. The absolute best cancer memoirs by journalists are therefore powerful, engaging and memorable but also quite distinct in style from other works.

One of the finest such memoirs is *C: Because cowards get cancer too* .... John Diamond was an immensely talented journalist and radio broadcaster with a regular newspaper column and a burgeoning career. In March 1997, he found a lump on his neck which was diagnosed as squamous cell carcinoma (a form of skin cancer). Cancer quickly took over his life. Following multiple operations and treatments he was left with no tongue, little voice and no sense of taste. He was also robbed of the joy of eating and forced to live on a liquid diet. At first, he was given a 92 per cent chance of a full cure. Despite achieving a remission, cancer recurred and hope of a cure faded. Within a relatively short period of time, and despite ghastly treatment experiences, the course of his disease went in an ominous direction and he was given a terminal prognosis.

The decision to explore the cancer world in his newspaper column came about naturally. His brief from The Times was to write about the minutiae of domestic life. In the week of his diagnosis, Diamond felt that to write about anything other than cancer would be dishonest. So began a witty, intelligent, painful, funny and no-holds-barred chronicle of a cancer experience. It eventually led to the publication of *C*, and then a second book, *Snake oil and Other Preoccupations*, which was published posthumously. In writing about the period leading up to diagnosis he captures the insidious way in which cancer often presents and how fears mount.

> ... illness creeps up on you. Only in retrospect do you realise that you'd been ill all along.

Diamond touches on that sinking feeling when it dawns on the cancer sufferer that something dismissed as just an inconvenience is revealed to be a cancer symptom.

> But most worrying of all is the tiredness. Nobody has told me to worry about tiredness, but I know it to be a symptom ... (p.239)

> I'd gone in to be reassured that I was just being paranoid, that there was no swelling at all, that I was imagining it all. But by the time I'd

been palpated and then scanned, and then ultra-sounded, I realised they were taking it seriously ... (p.244)

Diamond gives voice to how a cancer diagnosis changes everything in a heartbeat and a new life of uncertainty and vulnerability becomes the norm.

> ... nobody receives a diagnosis of even the least invasive cancer with anything but fear and dread ... however good the prognosis sounds, it can only ever be equivocal and even the best-augured cancers can turn into fatal ones. (p.7)

> The problem with illness is that nothing is certain ... And all the time there are qualifiers: the probablys and the possiblys and the weasel statistics which are wonderfully accurate if you're a whole population and meaningless if you are just a single bloke ... (p.87)

Diamond is insightful about the devastating losses cancer brings, writing as he does from bitter experience. Key aspects of living and dying with cancer emerge as themes in his work. His antipathy for the language used about cancer is one rightly shared by many. It is the language of blame.

> For it leads to the idea of the survivor as personal hero – that only those who want to survive enough get through to the end, and the implied corollary that those who die are somehow lacking in moral fibre and the will to live.

He rails against the tyranny of positivity and cheerfulness that is so difficult for the cancer patient to withstand and so damaging in its impact.

> I'd come to the conclusion that whenever somebody told me how much good a positive attitude would do me, what they meant was how much easier a positive attitude would make it for them. Positivism meant we could all carry on as before.

He rejects the notion that cancer somehow makes you a different person or indeed is a transformative experience. He is also dismissive of the idea that cancer should be seen as a gift, bringing the cancer patient to a more engaged and meaningful way of living.

> I have learned a lot about myself in nine months and a lot about those around me. Much of that knowledge is useful, liberating even. But the bad outweighed the good a millionfold.

As he gets his journalistic chops around the world of alternative medicine and the anti-medical brigade, he tackles with real vigour a subject matter vital for both the physical and mental well-being of all cancer patients. Classifying the pushers of alternative medicine, he places them into two broad groups. The benign group who genuinely believe in what is being peddled and are motivated by a desire to help; and the malignant group, motivated solely by financial greed. He further sub-divides both groups into three: the religious; the alternative medicine enthusiasts; and finally, those who admit to knowing nothing about science or alternative medicine but who knew of someone who was cured by X remedy. Although he is amusing on this subject, he is also hard hitting and rational. He exposes and clarifies the real dangers for cancer patients in taking the alternative path.

There is so much to admire in Diamond's fiercely human account of his cancer experience. Even as he charts the terrifying progression of his illness, his dry wit and ability to make us laugh is ever present. His astute journalistic eye, cast over the medical literature and the alternative medicine world, is never less than illuminating. The sweet glimpses of Diamond's family life are as affecting and authentic as the inevitable moments of despair, panic, unhappiness, anger, and depression. We never really doubt Diamond's fortitude despite his title choice and the grim subject matter. Tangible throughout is the essence of a man blessed with charm, spirit and a zest for life that even his cancer experiences could not lessen. Diamond forges a strong rapport with the reader and delivers a memoir that is brimming with style, substance and emotional truth.

The Museum of Words:
A memoir of language, writing and mortality (2017)

Georgia Blain
(*Australian writer 1964–2016*)

As I began work on this collection, I set two basic ground rules. Firstly, to include only those works that I was absolutely passionate about sharing. Secondly, no author could appear twice. As my research advanced, adhering to these self-imposed rules seemed effortless. There was such a wealth of material across all categories. The problem I anticipated was whittling the selection down to my chosen limit of fifty. Until, that is, the work of two writers demanded that the first rule should always trump the second. Accordingly, both Georgia Blain's novel and her memoir feature. As you would expect from a cancer memoir, *Museum of Words* addresses illness, treatment and mortality. What the reader carries from its pages, however, and what makes this memoir so special, is profound love and gratitude brilliantly expressed. Blain has written a touching love letter to what matters most in her life, though it was a life awash with loss and grief. What counts is fourfold: her love for language, writing and reading; her strong emotional bonds with three women – mother, daughter, friend; her relationship with her partner; and the potent beauty to be found simply by embracing an ordinary life.

Blain was a prolific and acclaimed novelist, short story writer, essayist and journalist. She had worked as a lawyer for a time before focusing exclusively on her writing. In 2015 Blain became aware of a difficulty with her fluency with language. Aged just 50, she collapsed with a seizure and was diagnosed with glioblastoma multiforme – a highly malignant brain tumour situated in the language centre of her brain. A terminal prognosis, surgery and months of rehabilitation followed in quick succession. Blain's tragedy was compounded by what was happening in the lives of two women whom she loved dearly. Just two weeks before her diagnosis, her mother, Anne Deveson, had been moved into a nursing home suffering from advanced Alzheimer's disease. Her closest friend, the writer Rosie Scott, had received a similar brain cancer diagnosis and was losing the ability to communicate as death approached. Through this unimaginably tragic time Blain struggled to come to terms with it all. As she worked to recover her language skills and began to write while gruelling treatment progressed, she initially produced a series of monthly newspaper columns about living with cancer. Finding the need to shape her writing into neat, standalone pieces constraining, she changed course and began writing this memoir.

Make no mistake, Blain does not shy away from scrutinising the devastation that cancer is wreaking. She accepted the prognosis and understood that she was dying, the only question being when. It is heart-wrenching to read how she yearns for things to be different and to be able to write about anything other than her cancer experience. There is a sense of mourning for the books that will now never be written. She is unsparing in scrutinising her predicament and the moments of crisis are captured in deeply affecting language.

> When I heard his words, my hope sank again, leaden, right to the bottom of the ocean. I had felt strong and optimistic when I had walked into his clinic, but I walked out bowed down by the illness and by the knowledge that I will be ill until the day I die. The mental battle is extraordinary. I do well for weeks at a time, and then I come undone. I am on the brink of an abyss so dark and deep I cannot breathe, my head dizzy as I peer down, my legs unsteady, my body ready to topple over the edge. There is nothing anyone can say to haul me away. I have to do it myself, crawling back from the lip of the crater towards all that I love in life, while knowing that I have to loosen the grip of everything I hold most dear. I am not afraid of dying. What I am afraid of is saying goodbye.

At the very worst junctures she encapsulates her feelings with terse but movingly expressive language. Her words are all the more powerful for their succinctness.

> Sometimes I was awash with sorrow and grieving. Other times, there was a saturated hue, an intensity that I'd never felt before. I was leaving the world, crossing to the other side, never really being able to join the living again.

Blain refuses to dwell in the darkness of cancer, however. She chooses instead to write more broadly, focusing on the cornerstones of her life. As a consequence, this memoir is far less about illness and dying than it is a celebration of all that makes her life richly meaningful. Her primary focus is on language, writing and reading, which are at the core of her sense of self. All three prove to be invaluable buttresses in withstanding the horrors of cancer even as it threatens to take language from her.

> Writing was the only activity in which I could forget time, and when you forget time, you forget mortality. Now, more than ever, it is my lifeline. As I write, I forget I have a terminal illness, even though I am writing about language, knowing that my own is likely to be eroded by the illness that I have. I become so absorbed in words, every one of them, and the layering, the structure, the balance.

As Blain tries to make sense of mortality, she writes movingly about what drove her to produce a memoir. The redemptive power of language is beautifully described.

> Time and time again, writing is my lifeline, the rope that I use, inch by inch, word by word. It is the way in which I forget myself, even though I am writing about myself. Some days, I feel it is the means by which I am keeping myself alive ... I feel that there is an inextricable link between my capacity to put words on the page and my being alive. So long as I can keep spinning these tales, I will be spared; I will live to see another day.

Keen meditations on language, together with insights into her writing craft, are shared.

> Language is at the core of our being. The way in which we express ourselves is inextricably linked to who we are and how others see us … For me the line between fiction and life writing is never clear-cut. Each requires drawing on the self and distancing from the self … [It is] a fundamental urge to shape experience through language, to create art out of existence.

Blain's diagnosis impacts on her reading. Although she finds herself unable to engage with cancer memoirs, other works provide a much-needed escape from harsh realities. I felt a real sense of connection when I found that the Neapolitan novels by Elena Ferrante, which brought me deep comfort during my year of chemotherapy and follow-up treatment, were the very same works that Blain loved in the aftermath of her diagnosis.

Blain's acclaimed skill with language and narrative structure is somewhat diminished in this memoir – understandably so, given that the building blocks of her craft were being mercilessly eroded by cancer. Yet this in no way diminishes its power. In fact, it is all the more compelling for it. Blain not only describes her struggles to write but demonstrates cancer's cruel impact on what ends up on the page. Blain still manages to resist a linear narrative and brings the reader on a journey that seamlessly moves forward and back in time and intricately connects a wide range of subjects. The beauty of nature as the seasons change and her disease progresses is still captured in wonderfully lyrical prose using language that Blain describes as a "gorgeous paint box of so many hues".

Tenderness flows as she writes about her ever-changing but always loving relationships with the three women, all of whom shared Blain's passion for language. When she writes about motherhood and her adored teenage daughter, Odessa, the force of that love is palpable but also laced with the terrible grief of having to leave her. Blain's exploration of her relationship with her extraordinary mother – writer, broadcaster, filmmaker and mental health activist Anne Deveson – features strongly throughout. The shifting mother-daughter dynamic is beautifully captured as she writes about moments of anger, frustration, guilt, regret, and dependency. Blain also uncovers the rock-hard and unshakeable foundation of mutual love. The horrifying impact of Alzheimer's disease on that relationship is something many readers will relate to. The nature of female friendship is teased out as Blain writes about Rosie Scott, who started out as her writing mentor and became a part of her family. Both Anne and Rosie lose their ability to speak over the course of the memoir and all three women died within months of each other. Illness denied them the comfort of supporting each other as death approached. *The Museum of Words* is a tender celebration of female friendship and of three remarkably productive lives. It is also a tribute to Blain's beloved partner and daughter and, more generally, to a world she loved.

> We are all dying. We all should be living life appreciating the beauty of the ordinary. But so often we don't. And this is the eternal human paradox: the only way we can cope with our mortality is to ignore it, to live as though we have all the time in the world.

The Museum of Words is a clarion call for readers to consider life, with all its vicissitudes and uncertainties, a wonderful privilege not to be wasted. She ends this wise, unsentimental and deeply affecting memoir with these moving words of gratitude.

> This miniature is my life in words, and I have been so grateful for every minute of it.

In your face: one woman's encounter with cancer, doctors, nurses, machines, family, friends and a few enemies (2007)

Lia Mills

(Irish writer)

For me, Spring 2016 will forever be associated with feelings of vulnerability and foreboding. I had foolishly believed as I started chemotherapy that I would easily withstand the required six cycles. As treatment progressed however, my body seemed to be falling apart. I had always counted on my determination to carry me through but it could not alter even slightly what was happening. Chemotherapy was first suspended and then ended for good in April given my perilously low blood counts. I was hospitalised, fighting infection and receiving regular blood transfusions. Paralysing terror took hold at the thought that this abrupt end to treatment meant remission was highly unlikely. My body falling apart was one thing but finding my psychological and emotional strength crumbling was quite another. Making matters even worse was my struggle to read, through the helplessness and deep anxiety, something which had never happened to me before. As luck would have it, April is One Dublin One Book month, a reading initiative led by Dublin Public Libraries. The chosen author that Spring was Lia Mills, a writer whose work was new to me. Her novel *Fallen* pulled me out of my reading trough. It led me on to her cancer memoir which in turn brought me back to my lifeline of researching cancer literature. For that alone I owe Mills a debt of gratitude.

From the very first read, I felt that *In your face* was a perfect fit for this collection. My initial impression only strengthened over the years as many more memoirs passed through my hands. It is an extraordinary work that certainly delivers on the writer's stated intention of making a real contribution to the literature of cancer. She draws the reader right under the skin of her harrowing cancer experience. She reveals the complex physical and emotional repercussions of cancer and its treatment. Anne Enright perfectly described it as a "life-changing book". It is a work that will help readers reach a far better understanding of their own cancer experience.

Despite her family's health history, Lia Mills suffered a delayed diagnosis of mouth cancer as she did not fit the established profile. Because it was at an advanced stage, her prognosis was not good and radical surgery followed by radiotherapy were essential. Her use of the tidal metaphor perfectly captures the trauma of diagnosis.

> The tide of shock recedes and I take my place in the waiting room. I wonder if this is how the knowledge of a diagnosis like mine works, that it comes over you, then retreats while you get your bearings, then returns. An incoming tide doesn't flood in all at once with the force of a burst dam. It sends warning, each successive wave advancing a little further than the last until the tidal lands are flooded. Then the retreat begins. My tide of understanding is on the way in, but it's not fully here yet. High tide comes later.

Mills undergoes radical surgery which involves the removal of a large section of her cheek, part of her lower jaw, lymph nodes and some of her cheekbone. The all-too-familiar story then unfolds of setbacks, infections, pain, growing dependency, and weeks in hospital. There is an immediacy and honesty to her writing about the various turning points on the treatment path that is really powerful.

> Each shock is new. This post op state of sudden weakness, pain, vulnerability, need, is a stronger version of what I felt after the biopsy … I'm like a raw recruit who gets wounded during training.

The developing relationship between cancer patient and consultant/ medical team is brought to life as Mills moves through treatment. The crucial importance of self-advocacy is touched on. Communication difficulties created by a combination of difficult medical language and the cancer patient's vulnerable emotional and physical realities are teased out.

> And yet, for all my note-taking and lists of questions, I still forget to ask the crucial ones, or don't think of the one revealing piece of information that I need until after they've gone.

There is a consciousness of mortality throughout, and frustration too at just how difficult it is to capture such a profound experience in language.

> ... we talk about what you learn when mortality tugs at you. The weight of your past and how your concept of the future changes; what love becomes ... But when I really face the wall, the idea that I might die, I baulk and turn away. I wish I could write something meaningful and unforgettable about that – and in the light of that. I worry that I've let my mind soften and run, like butter.

No such difficulty for Mills when it comes to describing pain and fear.

> It's like the breakdown of personality through pain. You become childlike. You wail, and then drag yourself together to clean up, clear away, carry on – and soon enough you slip back into the shadow and the form of yourself and hope the rest will return later, when the coast is clear.

Mills never shies away from writing about the truly horrible realities of her treatment. Nor does she give any credence to the happy-clappy positivity that appears in so many sickly-sweet books about cancer. Instead, and with great skill, she uses humour to lighten the burden. There are many examples throughout but one in particular made me laugh out loud, perhaps best explained by my weakness for all things Italian.

> A tall Italian Doctor with long hair glides into the ward for rounds. His accent and manners are enticing. The ward freshens up, becomes

more feminine while he's there. "He's lovely," one woman says wistfully, looking at the door, "and look at the state of me."

The humour Mills employs works especially well because the reader knows instinctively that it is grounded in reality. She creates a sense of intimacy and strength and uses humour, often very subtly, as a buffer against harsh realities.

It is not humour, however, that proves to be her lifeline. Rather, like so many other writers, it is writing. In this she echoes other authors who found writing to be indispensable for both distancing from, and comprehending, their own cancer experience. Mills kept notebooks from the start, recording in real time not only what was happening but also how she was reacting emotionally and physically. The writing therefore has an intensity, a laconic honesty, a sharpness and a clarity that makes this memoir special. The reader feels an intimate connection with this writer that lingers.

As Mills recovers, she writes wonderfully well about what should happen next if you are lucky enough to be able to walk away after a cancer experience. Her sage advice includes paying attention to life; appreciating and taking pleasure in all that brings joy; finding work that makes you feel alive; and always holding, at some level, the hard-won awareness that life can change or end in a heartbeat. Deceptively simple but utterly brilliant counsel for all of us struggling with cancer. Her analogy of the hooked fish set free is such a perfect description that it will forever remain with me.

> I have reason to know that life is unpredictable, just as I know that it's a thrill, a miracle, a matter of luck. And we stumble along in our daily lives, oblivious. Just as well, or we'd get nothing done. But there's no harm in remembering from time to time. No harm at all in appreciating what we've been given and what we could so quickly, so perilously easily, lose. (p.65)

> This sheer pulsing pleasure I feel is a delight in being alive, in having a house to be alive in, a family to be alive with, and meaningful work to do – it's a slow but certain glow that liquifies and spreads. (p.240)

In your face merits the widest possible readership and will be appreciated for its fine lyrical prose, its honesty and its insights. Clever, and very welcome, moments of humour lighten up even the darkest moments. I must admit that it is also a relief to include a memoir that ends in recovery. Every person living with cancer shares with Mills that hope of being able to put the experience behind them and seize the opportunity to be alive and fully engaged in the world once again. The writer Paul Bailey captured that yearning for recovery in his book *Chapman's Odyssey*. His is an enchanting novel where the dying central character finds consolation in the company of his literary heroes. Lying in his hospital ward, Harry Chapman encapsulates that burning desire for release felt by every cancer patient in just two sentences. His four wants - to be out of hospital, out of bed, back in the world, and back fully to his old self - are utterly relatable. Mills completes her memoir with two equally powerful and deceptively simple sentences. However, in this instance, she is celebrating the sheer joy of release.

> I was on the right side of that microscope, looking at what was left of my tumour. And I was able to stand up and walk away, to leave it behind.

There is a shared sense of joyous celebration when any cancer patient manages to put cancer behind them. The reader leaves *In your face* feeling jubilant as Mills ends her memoir free to move on to a rich and meaningful life.

Mortality (2012)

Christopher Hitchens

(*English American writer 1949–2011*)

Grappling with the enigma of mortality when faced with a cancer diagnosis is inevitable. Valiant attempts have been made in many memoirs to reach an understanding of the meaning of life, of suffering and of death. Questions about belief and unbelief arise time and again. Writers have interrogated what and why they believe or disbelieve as they struggle to find meaning at this most traumatic moment in their lives. I went in search of memoirs that took dramatically opposing positions on these momentous questions. As fate would have it, two of the very finest works addressing belief and unbelief were published within one year of each other. One is by a relatively unknown poet – at least on this side of the Atlantic – and the second is by a well-known atheist.

Christopher Hitchens was a journalist, author, war correspondent, orator, critic, polemicist, legendary debater and public intellectual. A gifted but divisive figure, he first attracted international attention through his attacks on Mother Teresa and was one of the infamous "Four Horsemen" of the New Atheist movement (the other three being Richard Dawkins, Sam Harris and Daniel Dennett). His 2007 book *God is Not Great* sets out his case against religious faith and organised religions. In 2010, at the start of a publicity tour for his memoir *Hitch-22*, Hitchens collapsed suddenly. He was diagnosed with oesophageal cancer, the disease that had resulted in his father's death. Within nineteen months and despite undergoing cutting-edge treatment, he died in December 2011, aged sixty-two. Ever the consummate writer, he produced an exceptional cancer memoir in the short period of time from diagnosis to his death.

Mortality is a slim volume that traces the progress of his terminal cancer and consequently his forced engagement with death. Initially he was reluctant to record this last major life experience. When he finally did commit to doing so, he wrote with characteristic style, grace and mordant wit. His book consists of seven essays originally published in *Vanity Fair* magazine. An eighth chapter, written in his final days in hospital, is understandably disjointed and unfinished but demonstrates that he retained his intellectual curiosity and the fierce desire to write to the very end. A serious and astute work about his time of "living dyingly," as he called it, *Mortality* does not shy away from tough realities which resulted in great personal suffering, loss and regret. But what is most striking about *Mortality* is just how wonderfully readable it is.

Hitchens was famous as a creator of brilliant phrases and for his ability to boil down complex issues into short, beautifully constructed passages. *Mortality* is littered with such writing and readers will relish his skill while remaining conscious at all times of the intimacy and honesty at the heart of this memoir. As only great writers do, he captures the very essence of common cancer experiences. Rather than the popular and ingrained perception of the cancer patient battling the disease, Hitchens speaks of a reality of passivity and impotence. With characteristic artistry he shapes language to perfectly capture the sheer banality of living through cancer treatments and their dire effects. It is sobering to read Hitchens's description of the horrific impact of radiation treatment, despite receiving it in one of the most advanced cancer hospitals in the world.

In common with all who live with cancer he has to tolerate the rollercoaster of raised and then dashed hopes, not only from the latest round of test results but also as word filters through about clinical trials and cutting-edge treatments. It is clear that Hitchens's passion for life and his intense desire to survive kept him on this rollercoaster of hope. It's not surprising, given his ability to imbue language with meaning, that he mocks the language used by the medical world, or what he terms "tumortown", as both dull and difficult. He is scathing about the tyranny of positivity that cancer patients have to contend with. With his trademark skill with the barbed remark, he denigrates Randy Pausch's *The Last Lecture* and the treacly Disneyesque life lessons delivered by a dying man. Outlining some of the unwanted conversations – often barmy, but always upsetting – that he was subjected to, Hitchens proposes a cancer etiquette handbook. There is a fundamental truth beneath the humour which cancer patients will really appreciate. Hitchens captures perfectly another reality for all those who live with cancer. Unsolicited advice pours in for the cancer patient from do-gooders and well-wishers alike, replete with pointers to alternative medicine and miracle cures.

Whilst interrogating living and dying with cancer, Hitchens unsurprisingly devotes substantial space to a defence of his lifelong atheism and to well-reasoned, if old and long-rehearsed, arguments against prayer. He returns to the well-trodden path of unbelievers targeting not God as such, but organised religion. He ridicules the hypocrisy and greed of religious leaders and organised churches. His unbelief remains robust, unmoved by cancer and approaching death.

As Hitchens traces the progress of his cancer in his time of "living dyingly" the physical losses mount, death comes ever closer and his tone noticeably darkens. He contemplates the damage done to his voice and ponders further devastating losses ahead. This is a sobering yet inspiring work written with a clear-eyed and fierce intelligence. The reader will relish not only Hitchens's mastery of language but also his courage and honesty in daring to probe the toughest aspects of his time of "living dyingly". Hitchens retained his voice and his ability to write, which were central to his sense of his identity, to the very end. In so doing, he gifted readers with this brave and wonderfully readable cancer memoir.

My Bright Abyss:
Meditation of a Modern Believer (2013)

Christian Wiman
(American writer. Born 1966)

Memoir writing is as ubiquitous as cancer itself. Finding literary gold in this ever-growing mountain of published personal experiences is a real challenge. Christian Wiman's literary exploration of faith in the shadow of cancer is strikingly different. He tackles the timeless and complex spiritual questions so many of us struggle to even articulate for ourselves. For the reader grappling with their spirituality at a pivotal moment in their life, Wiman offers something rather precious and succeeds brilliantly in his stated aim:

> I wanted to write a book that might help someone who is at once as confused and certain about the source of life and consciousness as I am.

It may be a short memoir but don't be fooled. It is a challenging read that demands our full attention. Wiman mines his own spiritual struggles for meaningful insights that help make sense of life, of faith, of suffering and of mortality. The reader is offered the ripe fruits of many years of theological, philosophical and literary meditation about Christian faith in a series of short essays. Wiman brings a unique mix of gravitas, intellectual metal and poetic skill to bear. By the book's end, he somehow leaves the reader feeling lighter and freer.

THE BREATH OF CONSOLATION

It has been suggested that *My Bright Abyss* is not a cancer memoir at all, so different is it in structure and themes from other titles in the genre. It is in fact a hybrid work that defies simple classification. In addition, some critics have pointed out that it contains very little actual text about Wiman's cancer experience. This is a total failure of recognition. The shadow of cancer is in fact a vivid presence throughout.

> My cancer has waxed and waned, my prospects dimmed and brightened, but every act and thought have occurred in that shadow.

Wiman captures the essence of his personal cancer experience in just a handful of unsentimental and densely written passages strategically woven through this mosaic of essays. No more is needed.

> From the moment I learned I had cancer – on my thirty-ninth birthday, from a curt voice mail message – not only was the world not intensified, it was palpably attenuated … And long after the initial shock, I felt a maddening muffled quality to the world around me … At some point I realised that for all my literary talk of the piquancy and poignancy that mortality imparts to immediate experience, part of my enjoyment of life had always been an unconscious assumption of its continuity … Remove futurity from experience and you leach meaning from it just as surely as if you cut out a man's past.

The harsh realities of living through multiple cancer treatments are expressed succinctly but also with an intensity and power that only gifted poets bring to the written word.

> I have been in and out of treatment, in and out of hospital. I have had bones die and bowels fail; joints lock in my face and arms and legs, so that I could not eat, could not walk. I have filled my body with mingled mouse and human antibodies, cutting-edge small molecules, old-school chemotherapies eating into me like animate acids. I have passed through pain I could never have imagined, pain that seemed to incinerate all my thoughts of God and to leave me sitting there in the ashes, alone. I have been isolated even from my wife, though her love was constant, as was mine. I have come back, for now, even hungrier

for God, for *Christ*, for all the difficult bliss of this life I have been given. But there is great weariness too. And fear. And fury.

The essay 'Mortify Our Wolves' begins with a sobering and unsentimental description of a clinic experience that sends a shiver up the reader's spine. It is full of the terrible dread and absolute vulnerability that stalks every person living and dying with cancer.

> There comes a moan to the cancer clinic. There comes a sound so low and unvarying it seems hardly human, more a note the wind might strike off jags of rock and ice in some wasted place too remote for anyone to hear. We hear, and look up as one of the two attendants hurriedly wheeling something so shrunken it seems merely another rumple in the blanket, tubes travelling in and out of its impalpability, its only life this lifeless cry. The doors open soundlessly and the pall of sorrow goes flowing off into the annihilating brightness beyond. Then the doors close and we as one look down, not meeting each other's eyes, and wait.

Wiman's words encapsulate the fear and uncertainty that is so difficult to manage when living with any incurable cancer. It certainly resonated with my own experience.

> Years of treatments, abatements, hope, hell. I have a cancer that is as rare as it is unpredictable, 'smouldering' in some people for decades, turning others to quick tinder.

Lovers of literature in general and poetry in particular will be enthralled as Wiman contemplates life, suffering, mortality and faith through his poet's eye. He delves into the literary texts that inspire him and enables the reader to travel with him on his quest for spiritual understanding. Wiman shines new light on the spiritual aspects of much-loved literary works. So many literary giants appear including George Herbert, D.H. Lawrence, Robert Frost, Rainer Maria Rilke, Emily Dickinson, Sylvia Plath, Ted Hughes, Gerard Manley Hopkins and William Wordsworth. It is a particular joy to find Ireland's literary greats featuring in such a significant way. Wiman references Elizabeth Bowen, James Joyce, Samuel Beckett, W.B. Yeats, Seamus Heaney and Patrick Kavanagh. Part of the delight in reading *My Bright Abyss* comes from his fresh, erudite and always stimulating perspective on such a diverse body of literary work.

> What we call reality is conditioned by the limitations of our senses, and there is some other reality much larger and more complex than we are able to perceive. The effect I get from poets such as Seamus Heaney, Sylvia Plath, or Ted Hughes, is not of some mystical world, but of multiple dimensions within a single perception. They are not discovering the extraordinary within the ordinary. They are, for the briefest of instants, perceiving something of reality as it truly is.

My Bright Abyss starts and ends with a stanza by Wiman and features his own poetry throughout. It therefore serves as a fine introduction to his own work as a poet. It is my hope that many readers will seek out his poetry collections in consequence.

Were it not for the Irish poet and philosopher John O'Donohue I would have been a little at sea when Wiman turns to the intellectual side of Christianity. References to Meister Eckhart, Paul Tillich and Thomas Merton made sense to me largely because O'Donohue's words had prepared the ground. O'Donohue explored the existential mysteries that Wiman is scrutinising, and from that same intersection of philosophy, inclusive theology and poetry. Irish spiritual heritage certainly suggests that Irish readers will be especially open to, and fascinated by, Wiman's consideration of mysticism. *My Bright Abyss* is the work of a mystic whose acceptance of mystery and mystical experiences is unquestionable.

> I do think that much of any genuine Christian experience is mystical, which is to say that it is timeless, personal, and that it suggests an essential unity between man and God. But Christian mysticism is not *merely* timeless or personal. The supreme mystery of Christianity is the way in which freedom from time is the call of time, freedom from death the call of death.

Mysticism may be at the core of Wiman's Christianity but he is also, as he declares in the book's title, a *modern* believer. He is reluctant to tie spirituality to any one church or creed and is cynical about contemporary American churches. However, he also understands the importance of the framework that religion provides and is practical about the practice of faith. He suggests poetry as liturgy, stresses the importance of extended silences, and highlights the need to be open to learning from other religions. Wiman draws an interesting parallel between his intellectual approach to faith and the faith of his beloved grandmother and aunt. Their faith he describes as attentive, intuitive and totally in tune with life.

> God was almost instinctive in them, so woven into the textures of their lives that even their daily chores, accompanied by hymns hummed under their breath, had an air of easy devotion. I looked down on that unanguished faith at the time, but now, after living with my own vertiginous intensities for all these years, that quiet constancy is a disposition to which I aspire.

Readers will leave *My Bright Abyss* feeling enlightened and fortified by Wiman's perceptive consideration of faith and of the role that literature can play as we seek insight into our personal spiritual struggles. As a man of faith, and as a poet, his perspective is always that of the 'insider'. He concludes that there is meaning in pain, in suffering and in death. He powerfully conveys a sense of life and of hope that is consoling. It is such a relief to be spared the trite answers peddled in so many bestsellers by mediocre thinkers. For those of us living with cancer, wrestling with faith and belief, and seeking illumination, Wiman's memoir is a unique and invaluable spiritual and literary companion.

Memoir (2005)

John McGahern

(*Irish writer 1934–2006*)

2005 was something of a lost reading year for me. As Cavan County Librarian I had poured every ounce of my energy, creativity, knowledge and experience into delivery of an inspirational central library and civic space for the people of my home county. Construction was nearing completion during a year that was an intense and all-consuming professional time. Any semblance of a normal reading life had all but disappeared. Thankfully, the members of Cavan Library Reading Group ensured that I continued to read at least one book monthly during that frenetic time. Shortly after its publication, *Memoir* was chosen book of the month. A McGahern work was always a cause for celebration, but could the master of fiction prove master of a different genre? The answer was a resounding yes. Here was memoir writing at its absolute best.

At first glance McGahern's book may seem an odd choice for this collection. After all, the word cancer is barely used and there are none of the details of diagnosis, disease progression, treatment, recovery or decline that so often dominate cancer memoirs. A closer look however reveals its absolute relevance. In May 2014 I picked up *Memoir* again, looking forward to McGahern's exquisite command of language and his wonderful evocation of a place and people so familiar to me. My perspective had radically altered since that first reading however, reconfigured by a recent cancer diagnosis. I certainly still appreciated the beauty and deceptive simplicity of his writing and the emotional intensity with which he captures childhood experiences. But it was an altogether different aspect that now overshadowed all for me and that is McGahern's masterful contemplation of life and death. The loss of his young mother to cancer and the deep wound that loss inflicted on him lies at *Memoir*'s emotional heart. McGahern himself was diagnosed with cancer before starting *Memoir* and although it is never explicitly mentioned, it is clearly integral to *Memoir*'s philosophical tone.

> The world of dying is different. When well they may have sometimes wondered in momentary fear or idle apprehension what this time would bring, the shape it would take, whether by age or accident, stroke or cancer ... the list is long. Then, that blinding fear could be dismissed as idle introspection, an impairment to the constant alertness needed to answer all the demands of the day. Inevitably, the dreaded and discarded time arrives and has its own shape: suddenly the waitress pouring coffee at tables, the builder laying blocks, a girl opening a window, the men collecting refuse, belong to a world that went mostly unregarded when it was ours but now becomes a place of unobtainable happiness, in even the meanest of forms.

John McGahern is a giant of Irish literature whose lifetime's work consisted of six novels and four short story collections rooted in his childhood experiences and in his homeplace, the rural counties of Leitrim and Roscommon. *Memoir* was his final work and regarded by some as his finest. There is a continuity with the recurrent themes of his novels in his life story. Further light is shed on his central artistic concerns. Chief among them was the nature of small rural communities and family life, unchanged for decades since the formation of the state. McGahern's laser-like focus also exposed the horrors of patriarchal and church control, and the absence of even basic rights for women and children. Finally, the nature of damaged lives of quiet desperation brought about by chronic poverty and the absence of opportunities and choices is ever-present in his body of work.

It is not all darkness however. There is also beauty and joy to be found in McGahern's miniature world. The quiet splendour of a unique and unspoiled landscape is an enduring presence in his writing. Time and again McGahern celebrates the resilience of the human spirit and the refusal to kowtow to authority, noting with relish small victories when tyranny is circumvented. Through canny characterisation he brings to life the wit, humour and innate decency of local people. His writing always gently prods the reader to first consider and then appreciate the joy that comes from belonging to a sustaining community that is rich in traditions. Although firmly grounded in the local, this mix of interrelated themes gives his writing a universal appeal. McGahern's reputation has grown in stature since his death and his work is a popular subject for academic research. Nonetheless, I suspect that it is his sustained popularity with readers who recognise and adore the breath-taking quality of his writing that would please him most.

Memoir traces McGahern's life from his formative years as one of a growing family with a loving, educated and responsive teacher mother and a largely absent garda sergeant father. A breast cancer diagnosis resulted in the early death of his mother, traumatising nine-year-old McGahern. Ominously, it also placed him and his six younger siblings under the absolute control of a capricious and violent father. Years of terrifying abuse followed. Salvation was found initially through a love for the natural world. Then a love of reading developed into a passion for literature and, together with a sound education, led McGahern to a career as a writer. He not only survived but thrived and his works were published to great acclaim. Writing life took McGahern away from Ireland but eventually led him back to his childhood place. The circular journey home to Leitrim with his beloved second wife brought him peace and happiness amongst the people and in the place he loved wholeheartedly. The sense of homecoming, when life with all its vicissitudes is accepted without bitterness and where McGahern felt whole and complete, is exquisitely conveyed.

At the emotional heart of *Memoir* is the presence of his beloved mother, Susan McGahern. He was exceptionally close to her. She nurtured in him a love of nature and an appreciation for the instinctive decency, comfort and support to be found in their close rural community. Her unexplained disappearance when McGahern was only seven (for breast cancer surgery) was traumatising. Susan returned home and for a brief time and was able to teach again. Two more pregnancies followed which surely exacerbated her disease. When cancer returned it was terminal. Her death at forty-two was the pivotal moment in McGahern's young life. McGahern was torn from her side by a father who failed to even visit. Instead, he sent a lorry to collect the children and remove all of the furniture just days before her death. Told from the child's viewpoint, the helplessness and distress of a nine-year-old boy forced to leave his dying mother under such circumstances is harrowing.

Her eyes were fixed on my face; she seemed to be very tired. I bent to kiss her. She did not move. I was bewildered. Both Maggie and the nurse turned away. I tried to hurry. If I did not get away quickly I'd never be able to walk out of the room. I wanted to put my arms around the leg of the bed so that they wouldn't be able to drag me away and they'd be forced to leave me with her in the room forever. I went out the door, crossed the landing, went down the stairs and out into the blinding day ... I could not tear my eyes from the upstairs window.

With McGahern, silence is always full of meaning. He wisely leaves the reader to imagine how this young, loving mother was feeling as death approached. It is disturbing to think of a dying woman deprived of the presence of her children. Even worse, she would have understood all too well how their lives would be shaped by their father when she was no longer able to shield them. That knowledge can only have torn her apart. McGahern's description of the sounds of a dying young mother's home being cleared around her at the behest of a callous husband, as if she was no longer of any account, is chilling.

> The iron beds were left till last. The joints had rusted in the dampness and the sections would not pull apart. Bicycle oil and brute strength were tried. Neither worked. They started to beat the sections apart. The sound of the metal on iron rang out and the thin walls of the house shook in the beating. When the sections were finally separated, they fell with a light clang. (p.123)

> Those who are dying are marked not only by themselves but by the world they are losing. They have become the other people who die and threaten the illusion of endless continuity. Life goes on, but not for the dying, and this must be hidden, or obscured or denied. (p.116)

Torn from the light of his mother's presence, McGahern found himself plunged into dark, oppressive years with his father. As is evidenced by the recurrence of the theme of paternal abuse in his fiction, McGahern spent the rest of his life seeking to understand his father's volatile and violent nature. Readers never doubt the absolute truth in his account of terrifying episodes in a reign of terror. His revelations are all the more powerful for McGahern's trademark restraint in the telling. Indeed, his siblings considered McGahern's depiction of their father to be kind. The episodes of terrible violence tear at the reader's heart, as does the ever-present sense of looming threat in their daily lives. This is captured perfectly in his descriptions of normal family routines.

> Each day was closed by the Rosary. He knelt at the same place as he ate, placing a newspaper on the cement and resting his elbows on the table as he faced the big sideboard mirror … When all the prayers were ended, we went up to him one by one to where he sat on the chair and kissed him on the lips, "Goodnight Daddy". (Page 58)

> He never acknowledged the server or any of the small acts of service, but would erupt into complaint if there was a fault … When he wasn't eating from his plate, he stared straight ahead into the big mirror, chewing very slowly. At exactly nine he would go down to the dayroom, and the whole of the living room relaxed as soon as the dayroom door slammed shut. (p. 33)

That McGahern survived the terrible damage inflicted and found a pathway to salvation is a testament to his resilience but also to the power of his mother's legacy. He managed to hold onto a sense of her comforting presence and to what she had taught him of gentleness, love and finding joy in daily living. All that she had nurtured in him – a strong sense of place, love of community, a capacity to take pleasure in the natural world, an appreciation for learning – would prove critical to his development. When McGahern discovered books and reading, he found a means of escape and a route into his developing imagination which quickly translated into a craving for literature that would shape his life.

> There are no days more full in childhood than those days that are not lived at all, the days lost in a book … It's a strange and complete happiness when all sense of time is lost … I read voraciously at first, for nothing but pleasure that was both a recognition and discovery and sometimes a pure, unfathomable joy.

McGahern's love of literature was nourished by neighbours who generously provided him with open access to their library. This, together with the influence of an able English teacher, enabled him to develop a critical awareness of what constitutes good writing. As his education progressed to third level the pleasure of reading evolved into a desire to write and with it he found his purpose in life.

> In that one life of the mind the writer could live many lives and all of life. I had not the vaguest idea how books came into being, but the dream took hold, and held.

McGahern's descriptions of the people and physical environment of his home place results in pure poetry on the page. It is in this miniature world that he anchors his work. Peerless in his re-creation of place, the poor soil, lush hedges, colourful flowers, small fields and dark lakes, together with the simple houses and local characters, come alive. Love of place is inextricably bound up with love for the mother who first opened his eyes to its beauty. In *Memoir* McGahern conveys a more acute sense of that beauty, no doubt informed by his approaching death. In capturing its very essence, he immortalises it.

There is a richly meditative quality to his writing as he probes his personal life experiences and the deeply painful childhood that shaped him. The understanding he reaches about the purpose of life comes from the pleasurable memories of walking the lanes as a happy child with his beloved mother.

> I am sure it is from those days that I take the belief that the best of life is lived quietly, where nothing happens but our calm journey through the day, where change is imperceptible and the precious life is everything.

Memoir is an emotionally powerful meditation on the transience of life, what gives life meaning, the nature of love, and how best to live given the inevitability of death. Read *Memoir* and you will be moved and consoled in equal measure.

> We grow into an understanding of the world gradually. Much of what we come to know is far from comforting, that each day brings us closer to the inevitable hour when all will be darkness again, but even that knowledge is power and all understanding is joy, even in the face of dread, and cannot be taken from us until everything is. We grow into a love of the world, a love that is all the more precious and poignant because the great joy of which we are but a particle is lost almost as soon as it is gathered.

PART 2

Novels

Introduction

As I set to work on selecting great novels about cancer that offer the reader solace and sustenance, memories of how and why I fell in love with the fictional world surfaced. I first learned about the power of books from my father. As if by osmosis, I absorbed both his love of reading and the pleasure he found in the physicality of books. I quickly became a greedy reader and can still recall the rush of excitement generated by my first library card. Our local library might have been tiny, but it was run by an extraordinary community activist. For decades, Caitríona Bean Uí Raghallaigh nurtured a culture of reading and learning in my hometown, influencing generations. How lucky I was to have my earliest impression of the role of a local librarian shaped by this powerhouse of community endeavour. I hope I honoured her in some small way in my efforts to make a difference as Cavan County Librarian. I know that she would have cheered me on as I set out to research, write and finally get this work published, despite all the obstacles.

From childhood on, novels that I connected with intensely helped shape the person that I have become. It was through fiction that I first began to make sense of the world around me. I soon discovered that real truths are often revealed through the fictional world. Reading sparked my consciousness of injustice and my growing awareness of how Irish social norms imposed stifling limits on women. Long before I heard the word feminist or learned of the second-wave Irish feminists who were challenging the status quo, it was the fictional world that awakened me to the reality that Irish women had few of the rights and freedoms taken for granted by men. Novels helped me perceive injustice and prompted me to think critically about life and oppressive social norms. Reading gave me a sense of a world of boundless possibilities and both the hope and expectation that such possibilities would open to me. Fiction suggested that the freedom to forge my own path had to be fought for. In short, my passion for fiction played a major role in my real education.

It wasn't simply a love of books that prompted my choice of librarianship as a career. I started working in libraries more by accident than design but quickly realised that it was the perfect fit. It is, as the inspirational American librarian Althea Warren once stated, a vocation without regrets that moulds librarians into becoming "givers rather than grabbers". Honesty, love of humanity, intellectual curiosity and a sense of fun are four essential traits of our profession. So how could I resist the call? A growing awareness of the public library as a physical sanctuary that can play a unique and precious role in the lives of individuals and communities sealed the deal. I felt at home working for a service that is such a force for social good. Promoting libraries, reading and literature is joyful work. It enabled me to support inclusivity and fight inequality in so many innovative and unexpectedly creative ways as my career progressed. Although the public library service went through transformative change over my career, its fundamental role remained constant. Playing my part in that role of connecting books and readers was an extraordinary privilege. Recently I was struck by a speech given by Althea Warren at a 1935 American Library Association event in Portland, Oregon which rings as true today as it did back in the 1930s. She stated that librarians must:

> Read as a drunkard drinks or as a bird sings or a cat sleeps or a dog responds to an invitation to go walking, not from conscience or training, but because they'd rather do it than anything else in the world. (From *The Library Book* by Susan Orlean, 2018)

The world of cancer fiction was a new departure for me. I discovered so many wonderful novels but also encountered my fair share of works replete with simplistic language and trite conclusions. The final ten choices have an international flavour. Australian, American, South African, Venezuelan, and Irish writers sit side by side. The earliest was published in 1961 and the most recent appeared in August 2020. Included are a Booker prize-winner, a debut novel by a fresh new voice, and a largely forgotten work, long out of print. All explore the cancer experience from a variety of perspectives including that of the person living and dying with cancer, the caregiver, the family member, and the friend. The shared focus is of course on cancer and mortality, but the styles, stories and characters are as varied as the writers themselves. The common denominator is writing with a touch of genius that brilliantly explores the bleakest human experiences with cancer.

The Blood of the Lamb (1961)

Peter De Vries

(American writer 1910–1993)

Market forces in the book world work to keep the reader's eye forever on the next big thing in publishing. As a librarian I have always resisted such efforts, believing that the world of literature has a richness well beyond the contemporary just waiting to be mined and, when treasures are found, shared. Discovering wonderful writers now largely forgotten is a special delight. Peter De Vries is one such writer whose work was once celebrated by literary giants including Harper Lee, Anthony Burgess and Kingsley Amis. By the 1990s, however, his novels were out of print and he had all but disappeared from the literary landscape. And yet, references to *The Blood of the Lamb* kept cropping up in my research. Considered De Vries's masterpiece, it is an absolutely compelling read.

The Blood of the Lamb, narrated by its protagonist, Don Wanderhope, tells the story of his life from childhood in Chicago to marriage and parenthood. There is a farcical aspect at first to Wanderhope's tale of bad fortune. Starting with the death of his adored elder brother, a series of personal tragedies unfolds. Don develops tuberculosis and is sent to a sanatorium where he falls in love with a patient who subsequently dies. His father ends up in a mental institution. Don marries an unstable woman who commits suicide. He relishes parenthood but the very worst tragedy imaginable happens when his eleven-year-old daughter is diagnosed with leukaemia, goes through the agony of the rudimentary treatments of that time, and dies. De Vries's masterful writing steers well clear of cheap sentimentality. De Vries lost his own daughter to leukaemia, so it is not surprising that he delivers a wholly convincing and mercilessly honest account of parental love, tenderness, rage, growing desperation, grief, and finally desolation. Unexpectedly, the reader also gets humour and wit in abundance. There are laugh-out-loud moments throughout that in the hands of De Vries, celebrated for his comedic writing, are brilliantly integrated into the story and a welcome relief from the intensity of the unfolding tragedy.

De Vries was renowned for attacking belief systems including those of religion and modern medicine. This novel abounds with clever and witty satirical challenges to both. When the young Don is discussing evolution with the family doctor he asks:

> "Would you accept a patient with gills and a tail – proving evolution?"
> "We turn no one away. Not even," Doc added, citing an even greater monstrosity, "when they can't pay."

His daughter's doctor glibly explains chemotherapy treatment and Don asks:

> "Do you believe in God as well as play at him?"

Don's musings get progressively darker, however, as his daughter's disease develops and his rage at what is happening grows.

> Among the parents and children, flung together in a hell of prolonged farewell, wandered forever the ministering vampires from Laboratory, sucking samples from bones and veins to see how went with each the enemy that had marked them all. And the doctors in their butchers' coats, who severed the limbs and gouged the brains and knifed the vitals where the demon variously dwelt, what did they think of these best fruits of ten million hours of dedicated toil?

Stein, a father of a child in the leukaemia ward, jeers at the hope of medical progress:

> "So death by leukaemia is now a local instead of an express. Same run, only a few more stops. But that's medicine, the art of prolonging disease…"

The first chapter delivers an astute but also hilarious dissection of religious beliefs. As the novel progresses his satirical swipes at religion become suffused with rage. De Vries turns the religious phrase "the blood of the lamb" from the Book of Revelation on its head and uses it as a reference to the blood of his own lamb, his innocent and beloved daughter with cancer coursing through her blood, blood which is spilt randomly and not to some great preordained plan. The slaughter of the innocent. While Don accepts that it is important to let people believe in God because it brings comfort, he concludes that neither religion nor philosophy can help. Repeated verbatim on two separate occasions, this paragraph outlines De Vries's conclusions on the meaning of life and its value.

> "I believe that man must learn to live without those consolations called religious, which his own intelligence must by now have told him belong to the childhood of the race. Philosophy can really give us nothing permanent to believe either; it is too rich in answers, each cancelling out the rest. The quest for meaning is foredoomed. Human life 'means' nothing. But that is not to say it is not worth living. What does a Debussy Arabesque 'mean', or a rainbow or a rose? A man delights in all of these, knowing himself to be no more – a wisp of music and a haze of dreams dissolving against the sun. Man has only his own two feet to stand on, his own human trinity to see him through: Reason, Courage and Grace. And the first plus the second equals the third."

De Vries reminds us of how precious and fragile life is and how we fail to appreciate it fully until catastrophe threatens. The rollercoaster of cancer treatment, with its remission highs and crushing relapse lows, makes for agonising reading. When Carol first falls ill nothing serious is initially found and the sense of relief is tangible.

> "The greatest experience open to man then is the recovery of the commonplace … Books to read without that shadow falling across the page. Carol curled up with one in her chair and I in mine … But you can multiply for yourself the list of pleasures to be extorted from Simple Things when the world has once again been restored to you."

When she is finally in remission, Don is permitted to bring Carol home and his observations are jarring but also darkly funny and desperately sad. After Carol's death from sepsis, De Vries creates an intense image of desolation, grief and anger with both God and fate. Don vents his uncontrollable fury by throwing a cake at the image of Jesus on the cross hanging outside a church. It is a powerful metaphor for the disintegrating and heartbroken self, exploding with rage and helplessness. We cannot fail to identify with Don as his anger pours out.

Don's reflection in the last line of the novel indicates that resilience can be found in compassion, for ourselves and for others, as we are all in the end united by loss. It is a final enduring image that lingers in the mind of the reader.

> "Again the throb of compassion rather than the breath of consolation: the recognition of how long, how long is the mourners' bench upon which we sit, arms linked in undeluded friendship, all of us, brief links, ourselves, in the eternal pity."

It may take a little effort to adjust to De Vries's writing style initially, but the reward is considerable. His sureness of touch and his ability to frame the tragic and the comic to such great effect is quite unique in the world of cancer fiction. Shortly after the death of his daughter De Vries managed to find some meaning in living by writing this novel. In so doing he produced a work so intense, so convincingly real, that is almost unbearable to read. And yet, it gives powerful voice to anyone struggling to articulate their own response to cancer and striving for meaning as death approaches.

Between a Wolf and a Dog (2016)

Georgia Blain

(*Australian writer 1964–2016*)

Finding *Between a Wolf and a Dog* was an exciting moment on my journey to uncover the finest cancer fiction. I knew on first reading that such a riveting novel was a rarity and had to be included. Everyone who loves literature and is struggling with cancer deserves to know about this outstanding work. Blain delivers a delicately layered narrative populated by superbly crafted and believable characters, all of whom are facing personal crises. At first glance, it might seem to be a straightforward story of a family facing tragedy. Do not be fooled. It is a complex novel that explores broader themes of family conflict, personal integrity, love, forgiveness, and human agony in its many guises. Looming over all is a terminal cancer diagnosis and the devastating knowledge that death is fast approaching.

Blain's interesting choice of title is a perfect fit for her chosen themes. A translation of a French expression "the hour between dog and wolf", it refers to the twilight time when it is difficult to discern the difference between the two animals, or perhaps between friend and foe, civilisation and barbarism, light and darkness, even life and death. Her title prompts the reader to consider how difficult it is to see clearly when disaster threatens, and when personal feelings and experiences cloud our judgement. The story revolves around Hilary, her two daughters, April and Esther, and Esther's estranged husband, Lawrence. Blain weaves this family's past into its present and in so doing exposes the fault lines and ordinary family strife that have shaped their lives.

The story unfolds around the central character of Hilary, who is a triumph of characterisation. The reader is wholly engaged as Blain exposes Hilary's inner life and the entangled lives of those around her. Hilary is not only grappling with a terminal brain cancer diagnosis but also struggling to address the estrangement between her two daughters. Blain skilfully reveals the depths of Hilary's struggles as she contemplates serious illness and approaching death. This is a female character with a richly creative working life as a filmmaker and an independent spirit who is in danger of being consumed by the crises she faces.

Blain communicates truths about the nature of living with and dying from cancer through the character of Hilary. She captures in words something known to every person who experiences cancer first-hand i.e., how cancer 'islands' you from everyone.

> It is almost too much, this increasing bombardment of the senses, each instant passing with a slowness that is pure and painful. It is as though her life has been in fast motion until now, racing forward, a great crush of people, places, moments, anger, joy, love, despair all coming to a sudden stop, colliding into each other at the gate, while she slips through, walking onwards, alone in a quiet land.

Those of us living with the disease know how cancer imbues our present with an acute awareness of the preciousness of life. Blain conveys this beautifully when Hilary is talking to her son-in-law, having taken the decision to commit suicide rather than face a horrible death.

> "You get a brief time, and it's so vivid and wonderful and not to be wasted, but of course you only know that when it's about to be snatched away. And then there's a fainter imprint left behind, a period in which you are remembered. After that you are gone."

Readers will relish Blain's skill in creating a strong atmosphere and in building mood. She uses rain as a powerful symbol. The narrative principally takes place over one day in Sydney when it rains unrelentingly. The rain is ever-present in the reader's consciousness, as it is in the consciousness of the characters. Rain symbolises the complexity of what is going on in the inner life of every character. It feels at times like Blain's whole world is crying in despair at terrible realities. There is a creeping sense of unease. Conversely, rain's cleansing and life-affirming qualities are also suggested. She reminds us that a day of incessant rain, just like a life in crisis, can appear dark, foreboding and devoid of hope. Yet it also holds within it the power to enrich and the possibility of growth and change.

This is an unsentimental and beautifully balanced novel. Despite the complexity of its structure and themes, it never fails to sweep the reader along, eager to discover what lies in wait for the central characters. It demands and rewards the reader's close attention. Blain's artistry in finding words to describe the oftentimes appalling realities of living and dying with cancer, and the struggle to work out what really matters as death approaches, resonates powerfully. That she herself was diagnosed with incurable brain cancer as she was editing this work is a terrible irony. Her subsequent early death was a tragedy not only for her family and friends but for the worldwide community of readers who love great writing.

Blain succeeds in shedding a sympathetic light on ordinary, flawed human beings coping with the most extraordinary challenges with grace and fortitude. The reader feels a kinship with this family and their messy, complicated lives that are so like our own. Despite having the darkest of themes, her novel is ultimately a joyous read that celebrates life's beauty whilst also acknowledging its fragility. It is a wonderful celebration of the human capacity to find redemption even under dire circumstances.

Age of Iron (1990)

J. M. Coetzee

(South African writer. Born 1940)

Living in this twenty-first century world it is hard not to despair. In Ireland, homelessness, health scandals, gross state ineptitude and growing social inequality are the norm. Wider world issues are even more alarming. The existential climate threat, the rise of autocracy, democracies under threat, endless wars and growing inequalities within and between nations all threaten our very survival. When we are dealing with cancer, striving to find meaning, and struggling to accomplish something of significance in the time left to us, it is difficult not to feel like we are drowning under it all, helpless and drained of hope for ourselves and for the generations to come. Until, that is, you pick up Coetzee's superlative though bleak novel *Age of Iron*. Despite its dark meditations on corruption, cruelty, illness and death, faith in life is renewed and a glimmer of hope is restored. Coetzee leaves the reader feeling that a positive way forward is possible for the individual through personal growth and that this may incrementally bring about meaningful change in the world. Life, however grim our circumstances, is never futile and holding onto our faith in humanity matters.

Coetzee's novel takes the form of a long letter from his central character, Mrs Curren (a white, elderly classics professor), to her daughter, who has fled apartheid-era South Africa for America. Mrs Curren chronicles not only the decaying of her own body under attack from cancer but also the violent death throes of apartheid. Like Solzhenitsyn, who identified cancer with the malignancy of Stalin's labour camps, Coetzee invites us to consider the link between Mrs Curren's cancer and the cancer that was apartheid. Always ideologically opposed to apartheid, Mrs Curren has lived until now somewhat insulated from and blind to the worst damage it has wrought. Through her relationship with her black maid, Florence, and Florence's family, she witnesses tragedy after tragedy including the burning of a black township and the discovery of the bullet-riddled body of Florence's son, Bheki. Bheki's activist friend is also killed, while hiding out in Mrs Curren's home, despite her desperate efforts to prevent his murder by the security forces. She is isolated by her illness, and it is another marginalised person, the homeless alcoholic Vercueil, who becomes her only companion. Their relationship, uneasy and uncomfortable at the start, becomes the means by which she successfully reassesses the value of her life and transcends her illness and death.

As the novel opens, we are led to decay and death immediately. We are brought into Mrs Curren's personal crisis of a terminal cancer diagnosis. What becomes apparent is that she is not seeking sympathy and her desire is to share life, not death. Despite having suicidal thoughts and feelings of shame, Mrs Curren, throughout the novel, manages to re-affirm the priceless value of life, even when it is being senselessly denied.

> "Such a good thing, life! Such a wonderful idea for God to have had! The best idea there has ever been. A gift, the most generous of gifts, renewing itself endlessly through the generations."

Maternal love is at the core of Mrs Curren's identity, but that love extends well beyond her daughter. She tries to support and save those around her, even those who are difficult to love such as Vercueil and Bheki's young activist friend, John.

> "When I lie in bed at night and stare into the black hole into which I am falling, all that keeps me sane is the thought of her. I say to myself: I have brought a child into the world, I have seen her to womanhood, I have seen her safely to a new life: that I have done, that can never be taken from me. That thought is the pillar I cling to when the storm hits me."

Coetzee's portrayal of South Africa under apartheid is one of a country regressing to an age of iron. It is an age where not only the country itself but also every adult, child, family and state apparatus are poisoned and corrupted, unable to listen or to feel compassion. Justice and any sense of community and humanity have been utterly corrupted. This is brilliantly portrayed in Mrs Curren's contact with her doctor. When he delivers her cancer diagnosis, but also later, as her cancer progresses, she is met with coldness and a total lack of empathy.

> "I wanted to say: I am tired, tired, tired unto death. *In manus tuas*: take me into your hands, care for me, or, if you cannot, do whatever is next best."

The poisonous impact of apartheid is keenly explored, especially in the descriptions of the "children of iron". Near the end of the novel, when Mrs Curren is assaulted under an overpass, it is by children who show no mercy. We see how not only the state soldiers, who are practically boys, but also the oppressed, have been utterly desensitised. After Vercueil is assaulted by Bheki and his activist friend, Mrs Curren intervenes:

> "He is not a rubbish person ... there are no rubbish people. We are all people together."

Descriptions of Mrs Curren's downward spiral as cancer takes hold and death approaches are deeply touching and utterly believable in the anguish they convey.

> "To have fallen pregnant with these growths, these cold, obscene swellings: to have carried and carried this brood beyond any natural term, unable to bear them, unable to sate their hunger ... Like insect eggs laid in the body of a host, now grown to grubs and implacably eating their host away ... *Me, mine*: words I shudder to write, yet true." (p.64)

> "The end comes galloping. I had not reckoned that as one goes downhill one goes faster and faster. I thought the whole road could be taken at an amble. Wrong, quite wrong." (p.140)

Particularly effective is Coetzee's creation of the character Vercueil, the alcoholic vagrant. It is a radical departure from how a caregiver is usually portrayed in novels and works brilliantly on so many levels. Initially it is Mrs Curren who, fearfully, takes on the caregiving role in the midst of her own suffering. By the end of the novel, she recognises that in fact Vercueil has been the means of her salvation. The roles of protector and caregiver have reversed over time, before finally merging into a shared one. It is a wonderful expression of what it is to be human. And it is Vercueil who is entrusted with her most precious legacy, her letter to her daughter. Writing is the way Mrs Curren comprehends and comes to terms with her illness and death, but it is also how she affirms her life and leaves her imprint on this world.

> "Death may indeed be the last great foe of writing, but writing is also the foe of death ..." (pp.115-116)

> "These words, as you read them, if you read them, enter you and draw breath again. They are, if you like, my way of living on." (p.131)

Mrs Curren speaks truths about tolerance and compassion. She addresses larger concerns about the degeneration of a society whilst also focusing on one individual's personal struggle to find meaning in life and in death. She is that rare, deeply moral fictional character – like Middlemarch's Dorothea – who will stay with me forever. Her refusal to be victimised, her desire to fully fathom what is going on not only in her heart but in her world, and her efforts to act on that understanding, despite the isolation that serious illness brings, are powerfully told. It is as if she is challenging us to figure out what is going on in our own societies and in ourselves and telling us that we too must speak up for the oppressed and the marginalised, whatever the cost. In saving others, Mrs Curren suggests, we are saving ourselves, and liberation is possible even if difficult. By the end of the novel, we have seen the brutalisation of individuals and of a society but also the transformative power of true compassion. Mrs Curren has come to terms with suffering, grief and loss. Her illness and death are transcended. *Age of Iron* is a wonderful example of the power of storytelling. In Coetzee's hands, a relentlessly bleak story somehow becomes life affirming, holding out the possibility of finding solace in the direst circumstances.

The Christmas Tree (1981)

Jennifer Johnston

(*Irish writer. Born 1930*)

I discovered Jennifer Johnston's works as a teenager and from the very first novel I was hooked. Here was an Irish writer of substance who would help me make sense of myself and the adult world I was entering. Her beautifully crafted, complex, yet always unaffected novels consistently enriched my life. Her practice of creating connections between her books simply adds to the pleasure of a Johnston novel. Reading *The Christmas Tree* over thirty years after my first encounter with it confirmed what I have long suspected. It has never been bettered as an exploration of the search for self-understanding and the compulsion to take stock as death approaches. A recurrent theme in fiction dealing with cancer is the struggle to make sense of life when facing an imminent death. In less skilful hands, this has resulted in many joyless, mawkish and ultimately depressing reads. John McGahern was right when he stated that no matter how depressing the material, if it becomes depressing to read the writer has failed. In Johnston's hands this theme is made comprehensible, compelling and somehow uplifting.

The Christmas Tree is the moving story of forty-five-year-old Constance, recently diagnosed with terminal cancer. A single mother with a young baby, she returns to her childhood home in Dublin to die. As death and Christmas approach, Constance takes stock of her life, her troubled relationships with her parents and her sister, and her failure to carve out a writing career. As she journeys inward and looks to her own past to make sense of her life, she is confronted with the elusive and unstable nature of mind and memory.

"I thought that the urgency of it all might make my mind clear. Show me a pattern of some sort. 'Depend upon it, Sir, when a man knows he is to be hanged in a fortnight, it concentrates his mind wonderfully.' One great saying proved wrong. I find myself lost in a forest of irrelevancies."

Instead of communicating with her sister or others around her, she re-connects with the ghost of her disapproving mother in a series of confrontations. My psyche responded with pleasure to Johnston's use of a ghost as a metaphor for memory, a device which appears frequently in Irish literature.

Johnston captures the distressing reality of dying from cancer. Her narrator, Constance, voices that reality convincingly:

"I am experiencing a speeding up of the ageing process, rushing through in six months the withering that normally takes fifteen or even twenty years. I am learning, but without time for adjustment, of the creeping incapacities of the body, the curious centralising of the mind on the past, the gradual withdrawal of yourself from the main current of the living, the pleasurable or distasteful contacts with other people, living people. I dwindle in front of my own eyes, unlike the normally ageing who only diminish in the eyes of others."

Johnston has always delivered powerful images of decay in her novels. Her description of Constance's experience of physical decay is both unemotional and believable. Constance's determination to deal with dying in her own way is utterly true to the way she has chosen to live her life. The reader longs for her to succeed in dying on her own terms and recognises the innate nobility of Constance's character.

The characterisation of Constance's sister Bibi widens the picture of Constance's life experiences and helps explain her determination to escape the world that her sister has embraced. Bibi is a product of both her upbringing and her unimaginative personality and stands in stark contrast to her sister. Bibi's tedious 'do good' instinct and her lack of understanding of and sensitivity to her dying sister's wishes is utterly authentic and results in some truly awful moments. Moments that many living with serious illness will recognise from their own lives.

As Constance narrates and records her memories, her journey inward slowly but surely brings her to a sense of herself and of the wider world around her.

With the wisdom and insight acquired in her search for understanding, she advises her old friend Bill (now her doctor) as follows:

> "I was so certain that it was possible, essential really, yes, essential to see the whole thing through on my own. I found out though that all I was doing was protecting myself against pain. I wasn't beating a trail. I never fought. I became very adept at keeping my head down. Here I am, eyeball to eyeball with death, and I haven't moved the world in any way. I haven't even left a footprint on its surface. Next week, perhaps, it will be as if I had never existed. How sad, a few people will say and that will be that. Oh golly, I sound self-pitying … I'm not … I'm just trying to say the truth. We're not given much to work on, are we? A few pieces of jigsaw puzzle and too little time. I would suggest that you stop taking the tonsils out of the rich and go and learn to live … learn to die really, because that's the only reality there is. Before it is too late."

The character of the servant Bridie, another Johnston female character who exists on the margins of society, is pivotal. Bridie's relationship with Constance is an unlikely but touching alliance. On Constance's death it is Bridie who takes over telling the end of Constance's story in her simple style. In so doing, Johnston subtly reminds us that all human life culminates in death, but life goes on and hope and joy are possible. A better future for Bridie and for Constance's baby is imagined. When an accomplished fiction writer of the stature of Jennifer Johnston tackles existential themes, the reader leaves her company feeling uplifted and consoled.

A Monster Calls (2011)

Patrick Ness

(American writer. Born 1971)

A generation of librarians educated in University College Dublin's Library School in the 1980s had their eyes opened to the importance of children's literature by Doctor Pat Donlon. I was one of many whom she inspired to read children's books with a critical eye as a prerequisite for working as a public librarian. Once my children's book reading habit was formed it grew over many years as did my appreciation for excellence in such writing. Little wonder then that *A Monster Calls* features in this collection. This novel transcends the age barrier and is as potent and meaningful for the adult reader as it is for teenagers. Strange now to remember how reluctant I was to read it when it was first published!

As an admirer of the work of the children's writer Siobhan Dowd I was aware that *A Monster Calls* should have been her fifth novel. She had created the outline and the characters and had written a beginning but died of cancer before she could develop the concept further. As Cavan County Librarian I championed Siobhan Dowd in late 2010 for a county-wide reading initiative called 'One Cavan, One Writer' with the aim of getting everyone talking about and reading her work. As the project took off and we received support from the Siobhan Dowd Trust in the U.K., I felt a growing sense of loyalty to her memory. Writer Patrick Ness had been assigned to finish *A Monster Calls*, but no writer could possibly do justice to Siobhan's concept in my eyes so I felt it was best avoided. That is, until the excitement around the book grew and it began chalking up stunning reviews and major book awards. I finally gave in and read it. I have no doubt that Siobhan herself would have applauded Ness for taking the seed she had sown and nurturing it into his own powerful narrative. In so doing he produced a powerful, gritty and intensely moving story about a boy facing up to the terrifying thought of losing a loving parent to cancer and dealing with overwhelming fear and grief.

When we meet Conor, the young protagonist of *A Monster Calls*, his life is falling apart. His mother is seriously ill with cancer. Support is nowhere to be found. Conor has a prickly, awkward relationship with his bossy grandmother. His dad has moved abroad with his new wife and baby and shows little interest. School is no haven as Conor is avoided by his classmates, pitied by his teachers, and the object of unwanted attention from school bullies, all of whom know that his mother is dying from cancer. Worst of all, Conor is plagued by a recurring nightmare. And then the monster calls, a wild, ancient beast of a yew tree that is intent on telling Conor three stories, but also warning that when the telling is done Conor himself must speak his own tale.

"Stories are the wildest things of all," the monster rumbled. "Stories chase and bite and hunt." (p.51)

"Stories are important," the monster said. "They can be more important than anything. If they carry the truth." (p.168)

Echoing the traditional folktales of our childhood, the monster proceeds to tell three parables. Unlike traditional folktales, however, the monster's stories are brimming with tough decisions, flawed characters and the messiness of real human lives wherein good and evil are not neatly delineated. The reader implicitly understands that the monster is in fact leading Conor to an acceptance of his mother's impending death. Ness captures in words the horror of Conor's emotional journey as he finally faces up to his fate. Jim Kay's powerfully evocative illustrations enhance the nightmarish quality of that journey. It is when Conor finally speaks his truth that we appreciate the searing honesty with which this story has been told. By having the monster stay close to Conor right to the very end of the story, Ness underlines how essential it is that children have an understanding presence with them right through the awful experience of losing a parent to cancer.

He took in a breath.

And, at last, he spoke the final and total truth.

"I don't want you to go," he said, the tears dropping from his eyes, slowly at first, then spilling like a river.

He leaned forward onto her bed and put his arm around her.
Holding her.
He knew it would come, and soon, maybe even this 12.07.
The moment she would slip from his grasp, no matter how tightly he held on.
But not this moment, the monster whispered, still close. *Not just yet.*
Conor held tightly onto his mother.
And by doing so, he could finally let her go.

A Monster Calls reminds us that great storytelling possesses power. It can enable us to process the horror, pain, grief and loss that cancer brings. It can help us to comprehend our emotions and so begin to master them. It is, in the truest sense, liberating.

The Spare Room (2008)

Helen Garner
(Australian writer. Born 1942)

In my ten-year search for great cancer literature one book would lead to another, and in some cases, many more. The build-up of titles and the somewhat arbitrary way in which they accumulated was usually pleasurable. Sometimes, however, especially when I had trudged through a plethora of poorly written books with treacly storylines so similar that they blended into one sticky whole, I'd begin to feel overwhelmed and close to giving up. Luckily, that was often the moment when a masterful work would somehow appear and reward my efforts. Helen Garner's *The Spare Room* is one such remarkable title. Compulsively readable and brutally honest, this autobiographical novel examines what happens when a loving friendship is tested to its limits by the heavy burden of dealing with end-stage cancer.

Drawing on her own experience of caring for a terminally ill friend, Garner places the caregiver at the novel's heart. Narrated by Helen, the novel opens as she awaits the arrival of Nicola, an old bohemian friend who is flying to Melbourne for a three-week programme of alternative treatments which she firmly believes will cure her advanced cancer. Flattered to be called upon to help, and full of compassion, Helen puts great thought into preparing her spare room and expects to cope with her friend's needs with ease. From the moment of Nicola's arrival, however, Helen grasps that her friend is not only dying but is also in complete denial of that reality.

"Her back was bowed right over, her neck straining as if under a heavy load. She was stripped of flesh, shuddering from head to foot like someone who has been out beyond the break too long in winter surf."

Yet, as Helen notes, Nicola is faking it – both with herself and with others – and giving "a tremendous performance of being alive". Helen's sadness gradually turns to rage as Nicola refuses to acknowledge what is happening and persists in believing that the crackpot treatments doled out by a high priced "quack" clinic will produce a miracle cure. Readers touched by cancer will relate to and applaud Helen when she expresses her desire to machine-gun those who profit from peddling quack cures.

Helen's duties as caregiver start to take over her life as the weeks go on. Her frustration grows with the all-consuming nature of caring for Nicola and the personal sacrifices she must make as a result. Washing endless sodden bedsheets, dealing with Nicola's agonising symptoms, and enduring sleepless nights and pointless drives to the bogus clinic wear Helen down to the point of utter exhaustion. Ugly feelings build up inside her that are exacerbated by Nicola's continuing self-deception. This alarms Helen and disturbs her sense of herself as a compassionate and loving friend.

"… but it was a matter of urgency that I should get to sleep before two, the hour at which the drought, the refugee camps, the dying planet, and all the faults and meannesses of my character would arrive to haunt me."

Helen longs for release and a return to her normal life. The reader senses that she herself is also in a form of denial and fearful of death. Helen and Nicola are locked together in a prison of unspoken truths. Both must find a way to admit to their fears. Helen needs to accept but also forgive her own all-too-human failures of compassion and mercy when faced with a burden too heavy to bear alone. Nicola in turn must concede that she is dying, turn away from bogus cures, and seek out legitimate treatment and the level of support that her friend cannot provide single-handedly. Helen tries to break down Nicola's flawed coping strategy and force her to drop her defences, stop denying reality and finally face up to her imminent death.

"Death will not be denied. To try is grandiose. It drives madness into the soul. It leaches out virtue. It injects poison into friendship and makes a mockery of love."

The tension building from the novel's start is resolved near the end of the three-week stay and sanity is restored. Helen's tough love approach finally breaks down Nicola's resistance. She abandons the crackpot treatments:

"It's good darling. Cutting off all that childish crap."

and finally admits:

"Death's at the end of this."

The limits of friendship have been revealed. Nicola returns to Sydney where she eventually dies peacefully, supported by her niece and a network of friends. The last line reveals, in characteristically subtle style, that Helen has found both peace and self-acceptance.

"It was the end of my watch, and I handed her over."

Garner builds understanding and compassion for her two flawed but credible characters as the story progresses. She shines a much-needed light on the crucial but often impossibly demanding role of the caregiver. The suffering it entails and the frailty of emotions it exposes are keenly observed. The darkest moments are unsparingly portrayed but are always delicately balanced with instants of tenderness, affection, dark humour and even flashes of simple joy. The disturbing nature of quack medicine and its capacity to inflict serious harm are laid bare. All in all, *The Spare Room* is a gripping and complex story of human suffering and struggle that reveals brutal truths about the cancer experience.

The Sickness (2010)

Alberto Barrera Tyszka
(Venezuelan writer. Born 1960)

Margaret Jull Costa
(British translator. Born 1949)

My love for foreign language novels is largely due to the influence of a childhood friend who lives in Spain. She has introduced me to many writers I would otherwise never have encountered. As someone who can only read in English, I have learned over the years that the quality of translation matters. Not only the writer but also the translator must be gifted. This is certainly true of *The Sickness*, a poetic Spanish novel by a Venezuelan writer with a powerful premise. A doctor has just received confirmation of his beloved father's terminal cancer diagnosis. Dr Andres Miranda struggles to find the right moment and, even more importantly, appropriate language to share this difficult news. This central narrative is accompanied by other strands beautifully woven into the plot. A hypochondriac starts to stalk the doctor, convinced that he may cure him. He manipulates the doctor's sympathetic secretary into responding by email but in the doctor's name. And there is the father's maid, who is struggling to keep her son safe in a dangerous environment.

Barrera Tyszka opens his novel by addressing a philosophical question.

> Why do we find it so hard to accept that life is pure chance? There is no cynicism in that question. It seems, rather, an expression of self-

compassion, a kindly prayer; a way of recognising the limits of medicine in the face of nature's infinite power or, which comes to the same thing, the limits of medicine in the face of illness's infinite power.

A key theme of the novel is the importance of language and how it can fail us when we are faced with the unyielding nature of serious illness.

> For the first time, it occurs to him that the illness might take away from himself and his father something he had never thought it would: conversation, the ability to talk to each other. The illness is destroying their words as well.

Andres considers the language he has used for years to inform patients of a terminal illness and ponders its inadequacies. He contemplates the professional language of doctors in the light of his father's diagnosis. It is a language that he now sees as pretentious, unbearable – and, even worse, useless when real communication is vital. Much of the tension, fear and claustrophobic atmosphere in the novel is generated by the doctor's failure to find *any* words with which to tell his father about his terminal diagnosis. Barrera Tyszka explores this failure of language with striking word choices such as:

> Andres has a hedgehog on his tongue. His throat fills with pineapple rind.

Language is disintegrating under the weight of grief and love and underlying fear. It is slowly but surely being destroyed by illness itself. Andres begins to question the rights and possible wrongs of sharing knowledge about serious illness. Does every patient need to know? Might it not be better for some to be left ignorant of their fate? In desperation, Andres travels with his father to an island rich in shared emotional meaning. Ostensibly this is a holiday but in fact it is the place where Andres hopes to find the courage and the words to calmly break the terrible news. Strained beyond endurance, it is no surprise that when he finally blurts the truth out Andres uses language awkwardly and at the worst emotional moment, thereby maximising distress.

> Andres could see that his eyes were wet with tears and that beneath those tears lay something resembling both melancholy and rancor,

some emotion for which the dictionary did not yet have a word.

Throughout the novel, Barrera Tyszka pays homage to other writers who have probed the nature of serious illness. The Peruvian writer Julio Ramon Ribeyro, quoted by Barrera Tyszka, brilliantly addresses the nature of physical pain and its impact.

> "Physical pain is the great regulator of our passions and ambitions. Its presence immediately neutralises all other desires apart from the desire for the pain to go away. This life that we reject because it seems to us boring, unfair, mediocre or absurd suddenly seems priceless: we accept it as it is, with all its defects, as long as it doesn't present itself to us in its vilest form – pain."

Barrera Tyszka describes how illness and pain can make even the strongest long for release.

> Death is preferable to pain. Illness is a very bitter toll to pay, a tax so capricious that it can make death the object of all our final desires.

A profound, philosophical exploration of the nature of illness unfolds. This beautifully paced narrative does not shy away from presenting complex characters, or moving in unexpected directions, but still keeps the reader fully engaged. Barrera Tyszka's exploration of how the stress of terminal cancer impacts on the tender and loving bond between a father and son is utterly convincing. This novel reminds us that, despite the horrors of serious illness, life is meaningful and can remain so in the face of grief, pain and even death.

So Much For That (2010)

Lionel Shriver
(American writer. Born 1957)

There is so much to admire in this absorbing, dryly humorous and unflinchingly honest novel. Memorable characters, a cracking plot and a surprisingly uplifting and satisfying ending are not commonly found in books about terminal cancer. The impact of serious illness on marriages, family relationships and friendships is explored. There is no doubt that Shriver's powerful and persuasive attack on the injustices of the American healthcare system results in some contrived dialogue and polemical diatribes at times, all delivered through a strong authorial voice. Yet Shriver somehow weaves those observations into a fast-paced, powerful narrative with outstanding characterisation. This novel is so much more than a treatise on the American healthcare system. Other serious issues are probed including the psychology of illness; the language surrounding cancer; the sad deficiencies in the way doctors, family and friends often relate to cancer patients; and the deep discontent that the rat race fosters in the human soul. Never sentimental, Shriver does not shy away from the gruesome realities of cancer, its treatment and the dying process. It is a work that is both believable and fearlessly honest in every detail. *So Much For That* is also brimming with unexpected tenderness and marital love. At its heart is a protagonist who is a splendid representation of the unsung heroes of the cancer world – the caregivers who quietly 'shepherd' their loved ones through cancer with little, if any, fanfare at all.

Set largely in New York, the novel opens with the central character, Shep Knacker, planning finally to leave the rat race behind. Despite fears about whether his wife and son will agree to move with him, he is determined to embark on a long-considered retirement plan, using his substantial nest egg to move to an island off the coast of Africa. After years of procrastinating, he is convinced that it is now or never. His plans for a better future crumble instantly upon learning that his wife, Glynis, has been diagnosed with a rare and aggressive cancer caused by exposure to asbestos. Her care will require Shep to utilise his savings and to continue to work at a job he hates to guarantee insurance cover. A parallel story unfolds centred around Shep and Glynis's close friends. Jackson and Carol are struggling to keep afloat whilst coping with a teenage daughter who was born with a rare degenerative disease and consequently faces a shortened lifetime, full of pain and suffering. The complex impact of serious illness on both marriages is uncovered layer by layer and forensically explored. Through the course of the novel other health issues arise including the need for end-of-life care for Shep's father and a botched surgery with tragic results for Jackson and his family. The difficult circumstances all of the characters face are subtly and cleverly developed and the ending delivers a moving resolution.

This novel shines for me in its portrayal of families and friends as they react to a cancer diagnosis. The standard image depicted in countless novels is of loved ones rallying around with an outpouring of unconditional support. Sadly, the experience of people living with cancer is often quite different and Shriver captures that reality brilliantly. Her creation of the selfish sister-in-law, Beryl, has been criticised as a caricature. In fact, she is a much-needed counterbalance to the sentimental tosh we are regularly exposed to and a necessary reminder of the many "Beryls" who populate the real world. Shep is initially shocked and then scathing in his observations about how family and friends disappear when Glynis needs them most.

> Beryl turned from the stove and creased her forehead, assuming an expression of deep worried solicitation, "How is she *doing*?" It was a look that Shep had learned to recognise. The very music of her question – drawn out, searching, dropped in pitch – was identical in timbre to the queries he'd fielded from ancillary characters for months now. Beneath the perfunctory, brow-furrowed performance lurked the hope that the answer not be awkward, that it not ask anything of them, and that most of all it would be short.

Some may doubt that the behaviour of Glynis's mother, sisters and friends has any grounding in reality. Actually, it mirrors a common experience and Shriver's portrayal crystallises that reality but also balances it beautifully with the character of Shep.

> Broadly, he'd been a little worried that, after stays of increasing duration, his sisters-in-law would get on his nerves ... Never in a million years had he expected to be contending with quite the opposite problem: that following that initial rush to his wife's bedside after her surgery, neither of her sisters would visit again ... With an acrid taste in his mouth, Shep sometimes recalled the fulsome offers of assistance with which friends and family had met the initial bad news ... Did these people remember having made those extravagant offers in the first flush of rash compassion?

The world of cancer is permeated with upbeat cancer rhetoric which perpetuates the myth that cancer is a battle that can be won if the patient has a positive attitude and a fighting spirit. Shriver demolishes that myth with precision. In so doing she frees us from the unrealistic and harmful impacts that flow from such rhetoric. In conversation with Glynis's doctor, Shep addresses the problem of the language of cancer:

> "*Struggle. Surmounting* the odds ... And then you guys jack up the stakes even more ... The *battle* against cancer. The *arsenal* at our disposal ... You make her think that there's something she has to do, to be a *good soldier, a real trooper*. So if she deteriorates anyway, then there's something she didn't do: she didn't show courage under fire. I know you mean well, but after all this military talk she now equates – dying – with dishonour. With failure. With personal failure."

Shep tries instead to help Glynis finally face the truth and accept that she is dying.

> "And then all this talk, at the hospital, about 'fighting'" and 'beating', and 'winning'... Cancer is not a 'battle'. Getting sicker is not a sign of weakness. And dying," he said the word softly but distinctly, "is not defeat."

Shriver does not stint on gritty detail as Glynis dies but she also manages to tenderly portray a dignified death, far removed from the horrors of treatment. Shep's dream of escape from the moral bankruptcy of his suburban life comes true in the unlikeliest if also quite American way. Glynis is watched over and cared for throughout the dying process simply and lovingly. Relish this terrifically readable and insightful novel, not least for its satisfying, if unexpected, ending.

Gain (1998)

Richard Powers

(American writer. Born 1957)

Approaching this novel was challenging at first as I was aware of Powers's reputation as a writer of fiercely intelligent but also difficult and dense work. Written on a grand scale and epic in its historical sweep, it is not a book that I expected to feature in this collection, nor even to like. How wrong I was. It is an exceptional portrayal of our complex capitalist and technological world and its destructive ecological and human impact. Never shrill or didactic, *Gain* is a thought-provoking and carefully considered work. Powers pulls no punches and refuses to deliver facile answers or indeed any sense of dramatic closure. Rather, he takes on the role of witness and trusts the reader to wrestle meaning from the facts portrayed. More than twenty years since it was written, *Gain* offers vital insights into what has brought us so close to ecological catastrophe with tragic implications for individuals and society – and in so doing alters how the reader looks at, and begins to understand, the complexity of cancer's causal factors. We leave *Gain* with a far better grasp of just how problematical the task of eradicating cancer truly is.

The book is composed of two narratives. The history of a large American Corporation is juxtaposed with the personal story of a 42-year-old woman who is dying from ovarian cancer. Laura's cancer experience, from diagnosis through treatment and on to her death, is unsparingly detailed but also sensitively and movingly captured. The hidden carcinogenic impact of unchecked corporate American growth is superbly drawn and the link between business growth and cancerous growth well made. The stage is set for the parallel narratives in the opening paragraph. The Calvinist roots of American capitalism are exposed as the town of Lacewood, home to both Laura and Clare International's headquarters, awakens.

> Day had a way of shaking Lacewood awake. Slapping it lightly, like a new born. Rubbing its wrists and reviving it. On warm mornings, you remembered: this is why we do things. Make hay, here, while the sun shines. Work for the night is coming. Work now, for there is no work in the place where you are going.

Powers charts the rise of Clare International from its early 19th-Century roots as a family business through every phase of American industrial, financial and labour development in the 19th and the 20th centuries. From its entrepreneurial beginnings in local artisan soap and candle production, the company moves to intensive industrial production and onto a global scale, creating a dizzyingly diverse range of chemical products with increasing ecological consequences. An intimate family business where all employees are known to the owners becomes progressively dehumanised and is transformed into a vast international conglomerate, isolated from human values and with shareholders enabled by incorporation to legally shirk their responsibilities. Powers's portrayal of Clare International's historical journey is believable throughout and utterly chilling.

The impressive story of Clare International's rise is tragically mirrored in Laura's descent into the harsh realities of living with and dying from ovarian cancer. She learns that it was quite likely caused by exposure to carcinogenic chemicals produced by the Clare plant. Laura's story is well told, perfectly capturing the horrors of diagnosis and treatment.

> She remembers bobbing up from the truth serum milkshake – thiopental sodium, fentanyl, tubocurarine, halothane – in a state perilously close to knowledge. The concoction left her with a continuous sense of micro-déjà vu. She heard the word 'cancer' a good two seconds before the surgeon pronounced it. Maybe it was still the drugs, but she found herself thinking, "All right. I can deal with this. I'm an adult." And for a second or two, she thought it might even be true. (pp.71-72)

Private confusion she might bear. But everything stays so plain, so ordinary. Standard order of business. That's the strangest thing about illness. Her body's betrayal changes nothing. The standing, routine pileup of diversions. How disorientating: here, now, all those weird familiars. Nobody sees, so regular is life. Nobody knows what's blossoming inside them. (p.85)

The reader is drawn into the story of cancer's impact not only on Laura but also on her family – her ex-husband turned caregiver, Don, and her two children. Laura and Don's gradual awakening to the reality of how their way of life has resulted in personal tragedy is poignantly conveyed. As the story unfolds, we witness Laura's fractious relationship with her ex-husband and her deepening concerns about her children's "buy in" to consumer culture. Ironically, cancer is the spur that makes her family whole again, drawn together by love but also by fear and anger. As Laura struggles to come to terms with what has happened to her husband, Don is determined to persuade her to join a lawsuit against Clare. Laura initially resists, recognising her own culpability.

> The newspapers, Don, the lawyers: everybody outraged at the offense. As if cancer just blew in the window. Well, if it did, it was an inside job. Some accomplice, opening the latch for it. She cannot sue the company for raiding her house. She brought them in, by choice, toted them in a shopping bag. And she'd do it all over again, given the choice. Would have to.

Powers powerfully communicates how cancer is entwined with chemistry and therefore with the chemical products we develop with scant regard for the carcinogenic impact not only of the production process but also of their domestic usage. Paradoxically, it is also chemistry, in the shape of chemotherapy and access to ground-breaking drugs, that offers Laura her only faint hope of survival. Powers raises our consciousness about how ubiquitous chemical products are in our everyday lives. On return from yet another hospital stay, Laura recognises that her vow to clear her house of Clare products is hopeless. Her life is so steeped in the products of corporations in general that extricating herself is virtually impossible. They underpin Laura's – and by extension our own – way of life.

Too many to purge them all. Every hour of her life depends on more corporations than she can count.

This is a novel with a rich and complex theme that is subtly yet systematically explored. The 'gain' of the corporate world is made by devastating destruction of the natural world. The 'gain' for society is in easy and cheap access to product, much of which we are schooled by clever marketing to crave or at a minimum to believe we need. We have allowed corporate culture to become an intrinsic part of our existence. The human failure to question this state of affairs has left us with a way of living that is dangerously at odds with a sustainable world. We have enabled this to happen precisely because we have not grasped, nor even sought to grasp, its terrible significance. The consequences of our complicity are far reaching and tragic. Loss is not only personal but societal. Extricating ourselves will require transformative change.

Gain delivers a well-judged and beautifully balanced interplay between a societal story and the 'dying' life of one individual. While the novel's central theme is brilliantly explored, characterisation is a little weak and the authorial voice dominates at its expense. Yet, on balance, *Gain*'s considerable merits far outweigh these minor quibbles. Important questions are raised, and not just for those of us living with cancer. Both the historical account of the rise of Clare International and the description of Laura's domestic tragedy hold the reader's interest. Laura's cancer story is placed in broad social and environmental contexts. The world portrayed by Powers is certainly not the world so often reflected in popular films and novels, where the individual wins out eventually and justice is served. *Gain* is grounded in a more complex truth and is a far more rewarding read as a result, albeit a deeply unsettling one.

As You Were (2020)

Elaine Feeney

(*Irish writer. Born 1979*)

My heart sank when news of Elaine Feeney's debut novel first reached me. Having completed the Novels section months previously, I had drawn a line in the sand and was determined not to consider any new publications. I had so much ongoing work to do that I held firm despite the growing buzz of excitement around *As You Were*. In any case, how likely was it that a debut novel could be good enough to take the spot of one of the ten superb novels already selected? I am forever grateful to a colleague whose persistent entreaties to *just read it* finally broke through my resistance.

There is so much to admire in Feeney's novel. A very modern mix of writing styles is used to tell a story that is sweeping in scope yet wonderfully intimate. *As You Were* is focused primarily on one week in the lives of three women sharing a Galway hospital ward and Feeney is note-perfect in her character development. The intergenerational women at the story's heart come alive and drive the story forward. We are drawn into the individual life stories of these complex, flawed but never less than engaging and relatable characters. Simultaneously, Feeney explores the myriad of ways in which women have been subjugated over the history of the Irish State. The toxic blend of secrecy, shame, guilt and silence that has irrevocably damaged generations of women's lives is uncovered. It is a rare pleasure to discover a novel that bridges the personal and the societal with such aplomb.

The central character in *As You Were* is Sinéad Hynes, a young mother and property developer from Galway who is struggling to come to terms with a terminal cancer diagnosis. For eight months, she has kept her diagnosis a secret from all, most especially from her husband and young sons, by spinning the lie that she is suffering from a stubborn respiratory infection. When, inevitably, a health crisis erupts, Sinead is rushed to hospital, but she continues to keep her family in the dark for much of the novel. The roots of Sinéad's ingrained habit of secrecy and her desperate need to keep herself closed off from others lie in the long shadow cast by an abusive father. In fragments of memory that intrude into her consciousness at critical moments, we learn of a childhood of unrelenting emotional and physical abuse. The understated, matter-of-fact words that Feeney employs to slowly build up a picture of that abuse tear at the heart.

> "I stopped reading. Years ago. When I was a kid and my mind was filled with Father, I needed books. Growing into an adult, I longed for them. There was nothing safer than fiction. But then I started out on my own, I was so busy. Books reminded me of all the shaking and screaming and suffocating and hitting. I couldn't concentrate on other people's stories."

Witnessing that level of brutality directed at her mother, too, has only deepened the trauma. The psychological damage wrought has left Sinéad with low self-esteem and an inability to build healthy, loving and open relationships. The pattern of retreating from pain and shutting people out is perhaps most poignantly shown in the nine-year silence that has followed the loss of a baby daughter in utero. Tellingly, Sinéad finds it easier to communicate with her husband by text rather than talking directly to him.

Finding herself in a six-bed ward, she is initially reluctant to engage yet, conversely, happy to observe her fellow patients, not least because it distracts from her own terrifyingly perilous state. The patients around her have their individual stories to tell. Margaret Rose Sherlock in the bed opposite her is recovering from a stroke. Motherhood is a recurring theme in *As You Were* and this working class, deeply religious "mammy matador" is determined to do right by her family. Over the course of the novel, she brings her serial adulterer husband to heel, for a while at least; arranges for a young unmarried daughter to travel to England for an abortion; and extricates that daughter from a relationship that promises nothing but disaster. In a striking analogy, Feeney compares Margaret Rose to a queen on a chessboard, able to move in any direction as she runs a family from her hospital bed. Next to Margaret Rose is Jane Lohan, a retired teacher in her 80s with a large family who never visit. She has dementia and swings without warning from brief periods of lucidity to moments of madness that can turn violent. The story of Jane's profoundly tragic past, like the stories of the other patients, emerges in fits and starts. The last two occupants on the ward are male. Shane, paralysed for years and largely unconscious throughout the novel, is now dying alone. Patrick Hegarty is a small-town politician with a murky past who has lung cancer. His cold and arrogant daughter, Claire, is a regular presence at his bedside. To this mix Feeney adds Australian nurse Molly Zane and Polish orderly Michal Piwaski who bring much needed warmth and humanity to healthcare on the ward.

As You Were is a novel that is deeply rooted in place. Galway's rural landscape, city streetscape, people and local dialect are all brought vividly to life. Feeney also mines the rich cultural vein of superstitions and religious practices with deeply pagan roots that persist in Ireland. She signals that intention from the get-go with a prologue entitled 'Pisreógs' and a reference to magpie folklore. When married with Feeney's incisive humour, these traditions deliver comic relief at key moments.

> Hegs had his share of soldiering Christian paraphernalia, scalpers, rosary beads, a bottle of Knock-Holy-Water, a photo of Padre Pio's mitten, and hanging over his head were a plethora of mass cards … Mass cards should be signed directly by a priest who adds the names of the sick to their mass intentions, but now they were often purchased in a local shop, stamped by the box-load by a savvy priest as he ate jelly beans in bed while watching *Sex and the City* repeats.

When Shane's health deteriorates, Margaret-Rose and Jane go in search of The Cure to Save Shane. As they await the arrival of the Holy Grail of cures from Navan, aka Padre Pio's mitten, desperate efforts to ward off death are required.

What makes this book such a perfect fit for this collection is Feeney's wholly authentic take on the cancer experience. There is such truth in her words. The reader intuitively grasps that this is a writer who has walked in the shoes of the seriously ill and endured the demons known only too well to those living with cancer. She lays bare the isolation, emotional distress, disquieting sense of vulnerability and growing dread that accompany serious illness. A case in point comes early in the novel.

> "Hospice is not an option. I can't be alone at night. The desperate hush-hush of weeping midnight terrifies me. There weren't *options*. I'd started panicking in the middle of the night, the brutality darkness brings, and waking lathered in that sticky sweat that turns cold and feeling a warm hand pressing down hard on my throat ..."

There is not one false step, from the moment of diagnosis on. Sinéad's desperate need but abject inability to talk about what she is going through is distressing.

> "I needed someone neutral, or entirely disinterested in me, to pour myself out to, to tell them how sometimes I felt a kind of loneliness with such a force that I needed to lie down, or vomit or take myself into the sea."

Feeney's tragicomic portrayal of life on a hospital ward is nothing less than a tour de force. She reveals the physical indignities; the loss of privacy; the shock of living cheek by jowl with a hodgepodge of strangers; and the systematic dehumanisation of the patient that is only partially mitigated by the empathy and compassion of individual staff. A bureaucratic and underfunded healthcare system indifferent to personal suffering is juxtaposed with the growing fellowship of patients trying desperately to keep their lives intact. In this strange, detached world of the seriously ill a sense of solidarity develops. Small kindnesses and meaningful support for one another make all the difference. These moments of interaction are never less than believable but always devoid of sentimentality. Feeney delivers a brilliant and unflinchingly honest portrayal of what it is like to be a seriously ill patient at the mercy of a paternalistic healthcare system. She portrays a sad reality that is far removed from the patient-centred model of care every human being deserves. This is seen most powerfully in her description of the doctors' rounds.

> "Suddenly like slaying spectators, numerous teams of doctors descended on our peace ... They shut my curtains around themselves ... Some head consultant arrived, late to the party ... Looking for bloods and age and occupation again, over and over again this diagnosis of my socio-economic situation ... He directed none of his questions to me ... He'd met me before. But forgotten. And before. Forgotten that time too... And Oncology came. And Respiratory

arrived. And a nice woman from Palliative Care popped her head in. And would pop her head in again. And then all went off and sat around a big table. At a Round Table Meeting. (Via email.) And decided what was best (for me/without me). But no one will ever tell me. What. To. Do. Ever. I didn't even get an email or seat at the table."

Sinéad learns that her cancer is metastasising and that it is vital to consider her options from a doctor whom she describes as talking whilst "staring at my knees".

"But look, in all honesty you can buy yourself time, Sinéad, maybe, if you just try to consider your options. But you know, it is ultimately up to you. I don't want to force the issue."

This stands in stark contrast to Margaret Rose's compassionate concern for Sinéad, shown in so many meaningful ways as the novel progresses.

Dark and depressing themes are explored in *As You Were* and yet it is a gloriously uplifting read, pulsating with life. It's not hard to see how Feeney achieved this. The answer lies in her sharply observant eye; a poetic voice that is suffused with dark humour and biting wit; and the layers of meaning crafted into the plot. Ultimately, though, it is the absolute authenticity of her writing about serious illness and mortality and the accomplished manner in which she captures the intensity of the cancer experience that clinches it for me.

PART 3

Poetry

Introduction

A curious thing happened following my cancer diagnosis. My reading life up until that moment had centred almost exclusively on the world of prose. I had never strayed too deeply into the poetry world although I did have favourite poets and indeed favourite poems. I always enjoyed dipping into poetry anthologies and dutifully read the work of the many visiting poets to the libraries where I worked over many years. Reading poetry seriously and extensively was a departure, however, and one that proved transformative. Over time, my ear gradually became more attuned to poetic language, the fear of failing to grasp meanings receded, my confidence grew and a door which had already been slightly ajar opened wide. I discovered that the skill of reading poetry can be developed with just a little more effort. The rewards are inestimable.

Poetry was the section that I dreaded most when it came to the selection process. In fact, it proved to be the easiest and, in many ways, the most pleasurable to do. If I had to choose just one literary genre as the ultimate medium for articulating the experience of cancer it would be poetry. The ten exceptional collections chosen are vivid evocations of the cancer experience. Plainly put, this is great poetry that gets to the very heart of the matter, crystallising tough experiences. Through this process, it helps us make sense of our own thoughts and feelings about serious illness and approaching death. We are reminded that we are not alone and what we are going through has been experienced by others.

Poetry written in the shadow of death and illuminating a world of immense suffering, uncertainty, dread, loss, helplessness, rage and grief may not seem at all enticing. Harrowing descriptions of cancer experiences and the painful search for deeper understanding does make for challenging reading. It is difficult to witness intense vulnerability and pain. Yet all of the ten poets I have included have such authentic and profound poetic voices that we are riveted. Giving voice to the complex truth of their own experience, they offer us a powerful and welcome reminder of humanity's shared fragility. Moreover, it is as if our own deepest concerns have finally been articulated. The themes are dark, of course, and there is a sense of foreboding like a throbbing vein running right through this section but, paradoxically, every single collection, without exception, is alive to the beauty of the world and the preciousness of life.

Each poet uses their masterly command of language and form to create work that is subtle and dense with meaning. The pleasure to be found in individual poems is intensified and enriched as emergent themes, images and meanings develop across a collection. Some of the collections are meticulously constructed, with a pace, a rhythm and a momentum that is irresistible. Wit, humour and a sense of irony are brilliantly used throughout. I particularly loved the killer, knife-twist endings employed so effectively by a number of the poets. As the major themes of cancer literature are explored, ideas do converge but they are communicated in each poet's unique style.

There are many points of connection between the collections beyond the obvious central themes of serious illness and mortality. The importance of the relationship with a life partner features heavily. A sense of place and a delight in natural landscapes are set against deep concerns about environmental destruction and the climate catastrophe. There is also a welcome reminder of natural and man-made patterns of regeneration and transformation. In responding to timeless questions about serious illness and mortality, all ten collections have a profoundly spiritual quality, with one poet focusing explicitly on the existence of God and the presence of faith. Predictably, with such diverse voices, a variety of forms and tones and a multiplicity of genres are revealed. The reader is spoilt for choice and will encounter poetry that is confessional, lyrical, ekphrastic, elegiac, georgic, pastoral, metaphorical, fantastical and spiritual. What all poets have in common besides a razor-sharp focus on cancer and mortality is the quality of their craft and the magnitude of their talent.

The seven male and three female poets selected created by far the finest cancer poetry I encountered over a ten-year research period. Literary giants feature. The Romanian poet Marin Sorescu was a nominee for the Nobel Prize in Literature. The U.S. Poet Laureate and respected academic Donald Hall was one of the leading American poets of his generation. Short story writer and poet Raymond Carver has grown in literary stature since his death in 1988. All three are writers of international standing, widely admired by their peers and loved by poetry lovers worldwide.

INTRODUCTION

Equally deserving of international respect and attention but perhaps less well known beyond their national, or in some cases continental, boundaries are poets Ciaran Carson, Helen Dunmore, Jo Shapcott, Christian Wiman and Philip Hodgins. Peers and critics within the poetry world hold their prize-winning collections in the highest esteem. Deservedly so. Poetry lovers will be familiar with some of their work. To those who chiefly read prose their names will be largely unfamiliar and their poetry unknown. My hope is that this collection will serve as a useful introduction and new readers will come to relish their breathtaking poetic voices.

Just two out of the ten poets await introduction. Clive James the television presenter, memoirist, novelist, essayist and literary critic is well known. However, Clive James the poet merits greater attention and the widest possible readership. *Sentenced to Life* is a revelation. Like Ciaran Carson's *Still Life*, it does not shrink from the harsh realities of the cancer experience but has a life-affirming quality and a tone of hard-won acceptance that is deeply consoling. This introduction was destined to end with the American poet Mary Bradish O'Connor. Firstly, I wanted to honour some of the wonderful poetry that never features on prize lists or in literary reviews and very often sits neglected on bookshop and library shelves across the world. It is largely forgotten but always ripe for discovery. *Say Yes Quickly* is one such collection. It had a profound impact on me personally, not least because I first encountered O'Connor's work whilst in the chemotherapy chair. I was awed by how accomplished her poetry is and how strongly connected I felt to her work. Like Helen Dunmore and Jo Shapcott, O'Connor's powerful poetic voice and perceptive poetry is rooted in the woman's perspective. She is alive to, and engaged with, the world beyond serious illness. The reader senses her determination to embrace every last moment. She is a prime example of a poet who deserves to be widely read and loved.

The sheer joy of reading great poetry became real for me as I intensively explored it for the first time in my life. I discovered that an academic passport is not a requirement and that there is absolutely no need to feel intimidated by the world of poetry. Without consciously realising it at first, I fell in love with poetry and crossed the Rubicon into an infinitely richer reading life. For this I am forever grateful. My hope is that readers will share my delight in the collective force of the ten remarkable poets who gifted us such matchless and diverse poetry collections about cancer and mortality.

Sentenced to Life:
Poems 2011–2014 (2015)

Clive James

(Australian writer 1939–2019)

Unlike many of my generation who knew Clive James primarily as a television presenter, my earliest encounter was with Clive James the writer. Boarding school followed by years living in rented accommodation severely limited my television exposure. In hindsight I can see that this was a godsend for my reading life. James's humour and ease with words in *Unreliable Memoirs* first caught my interest. I quickly became addicted not only to his writing but, albeit belatedly, to his television presence. His appeal was manifold. His absolute relish for words, spoken and written, sprang from both the television screen and the printed page. He had a unique and unfailing ability to bring humour not just to the lightest of matters but, just as adroitly, to more serious concerns. A rare capacity to move seamlessly, often playfully, between lowbrow and highbrow subjects was part of his appeal. Clive James clearly shared the public librarian's ethos that literature and the arts are for everyone to appreciate, understand and enjoy. A learned man, he wore that scholarship lightly and was never pompous, preachy or elitist in his approach. Both in writing and on screen, he had an uncanny ability to make readers and viewers feel like he was speaking directly to them. A gifted communicator, he brought lucidity to any subject that captured his attention and always managed to get right to the heart of the matter. His huge appetite for everything life has to offer and the pleasure he took in life's absurdities was irresistible. It was impossible not to be charmed by his brilliance as a raconteur. The Irish soul is particularly susceptible to being seduced by this skill, steeped in a rich oral and written storytelling tradition as we are. In addition, buried deep in the Irish psyche is the emigrant experience and the complex nature of the emigrant's relationship with the home country. Irish readers are therefore particularly sensitive to James's love for his home country, a love that is reflected in the many poignant and wistful references to Australia scattered throughout his body of work.

Although rightly appreciated for his humour and exuberance, James was deadly serious about the importance of books and reading. He dedicated much of his life not only to appraising but also to producing literature. Over the years, I read his novels, memoirs, essays and television criticism. Yet somehow Clive James the poet never really registered. Until, that is, I started work on this book. A few short months after my diagnosis with Chronic Lymphocytic Leukaemia – coincidentally the form of leukaemia that James lived with – I stumbled upon his poem 'Japanese Maple'. So beautiful it almost stopped my heart, I loved it instantly. For me, it conveys exactly how it feels to be living with cancer and in the shadow of death and yet somehow more intensely alive than ever before to the beauty of this world. Sorrowful, wise, suffused with gratitude for life's beauty and emotionally affecting, it touched a chord at a vulnerable moment in my life that has reverberated ever since. It now has a permanent home in my heart.

When *Sentenced to Life* appeared in 2015, 'Japanese Maple' was joined by thirty-six new poems in one slim but thrilling volume. James's ease with rhyme and the musicality of his poetry did not surprise, yet the immense craft visible throughout was unexpected. This wonderfully accessible collection is the work of a man who clearly was a born poet. There is no mistaking James's distinctive voice nor the sheer accessibility of his poetry. (The punning title is so James-esque it made me chuckle as I picked the book up for the first time. It is a vivid reminder of the delight he took in playing with words and meaning.) Yet there is also a subtlety and a complexity here that rewards the reader with every re-reading. Although countless poetry collections passed through my hands, including James's fine last collection *Injury Time*, *Sentenced to Life* has established itself as a firm favourite.

Described by James himself as his "funeral" poems, this collection is a clear-eyed, unsentimental and unflinchingly honest exploration of mortality and human frailty. He invites us to join him on his personal journey of self-discovery and he reveals his vulnerabilities with real courage. His narrative style makes it especially appealing for readers for whom prose, not poetry, is a more natural fit. Many of the difficult questions familiar to people living with cancer are raised. What have I done with my life? Have I achieved anything of real value? Where is the real meaning in my life to be found? What is the purpose of my existence and am I fulfilling that purpose? How best am I to live now, knowing that serious illness is my only reality? Is it ever too late to learn about yourself and be true to who you are? As he addresses these questions, James openly grapples with guilt and regret as he humbly acknowledges his past sins and admits his remorse. There is an emotional depth to the confessional aspect of this collection that is deeply affecting.

Sentenced to Life is awash with phrases and images that linger in the reader's mind. He perfectly captures the harsh realities of living with a failing body and facing up to imminent death. The emigrant's yearning for the landscape of home, to which he knows he will never return but is forever alive in his imagination, is particularly poignant. Yet, what seems at first glance to be purely elegiac verse transforms on closer reading into wonderful love poetry. There is an outpouring of love and gratitude for a world that has blessed him with so much richness. He celebrates the natural world, close and loving relationships, family, and the sweetness and preciousness of life. The defining tone of this collection, which makes it so appropriate for people living with cancer, is one of hard-won acceptance – self-acceptance and acceptance of the transience of an individual's life. As difficult as it is, coming to accept his death is made easier by the deep comfort James finds in knowing that life, with all its boundless possibilities, will continue after he has gone.

These remarkable poems have been my staunch companions through difficult times. Seek out the shelter of James's writing. It is neither bleak nor depressing. For work that deals so robustly with human frailty and death, it is surprisingly life-affirming and is suffused with a hard-won peace. Clive James had a glorious voice that was unlike any other. Facing death only energised that voice and resulted in some of the wisest and finest poetry that you will ever encounter.

Elementary Sonnet

Tired out from getting up and getting dressed
I lie down for a while to get some rest,
And so begins another day of not
Achieving much except to dent the cot
For just the depth appropriate to my weight –
Which is no chasm, in my present state.
By rights my feet should barely touch the floor
And yet my legs are heavy metal. More
And more I sit down to write less and less,
Taking a half hour's break from helplessness
To craft a single stanza meant to give
Thanks for the heartbeat which still lets me live:
A consolation even now, so late –
When soon my poor bed will be smooth and straight.

Inside the Wave *from* Counting Backwards: Poems 1975–2017

Helen Dunmore

(English writer 1952–2017)

Helen Dunmore's *Inside the Wave* perfectly illustrates how reading poems as a collection creates a rich and rewarding experience. It contains individual poems that are compelling when read alone. When all forty-eight poems are read together, however, a more profound reading experience results, showing that the whole is so much greater than the sum of its parts. Shifts in mood and message occur within individual poems but also across poems. Themes appear and re-appear and poems frequently echo and amplify each other. It is as if the clarity of the poet's voice rings out more purely as each poem is read and understood within the context of the poems gathered around it. By the end, the reader feels connected to and consoled by what Helen Dunmore has to say about living with a terminal cancer diagnosis. The beauty and authenticity of this collection by a writer at the zenith of her career gives it a broad appeal but it has special meaning for those of us living and dying with cancer.

Helen Dunmore was one of those rare writers who moved easily and successfully between literary genres. Her body of work is impressive in its consistent quality and range. A prolific writer, she was and is widely admired as a novelist, a poet, a children's writer, a young adult writer, a short story writer and a critic. She was listed for, or won, many of the major literary awards including the McKitterick Prize, the Orange Prize, the Man Booker Prize, the Walter

Scott Prize, the Impac Award and the Whitbread/Costa Award. A dedicated coterie of readers awaited each new publication with high expectations.

Although some critics speak of Dunmore as having begun and ended her career as a poet, she is unmistakably a poet in every genre she wrote in. I first discovered her through a love of historical fiction. In writing her novels, she frequently used tools drawn from a poet's arsenal, such as the use of lyrical and sensorially rich language. She also demonstrated great confidence and skill in showing not telling, gifting the reader an active role in constructing story and meaning. A poet's power is evident in her descriptive and atmospheric writing. Reading her last novel, *Birdcage Walk*, I was saddened to discover from the afterword that a writer whose work I had long loved was seriously ill. *Inside the Wave* was published one month after *Birdcage Walk* and very shortly before her death.

The central theme of *Inside the Wave* is mortality and the experience of being poised on a threshold between the living world and the unknown as death fast approaches. Sub-themes emerge as she explores the transient nature of life and how time is experienced in multiple ways. Dunmore expresses fundamental truths about the meaning and value of what we leave behind. References to Greek literature and mythology in a number of poems enrich her reflections on the difficulties of facing death and dealing with uncertainty and dread. It is a fitting reminder of the timeless and universal nature of the human struggle to understand the process of dying and death itself. Dunmore commandeers poems by the Latin poet Catullus. Readers unfamiliar with Greek and Roman literature should have no concerns, however. She skilfully recasts these poems to broaden and deepen her imaginative approach to her chosen themes, making something altogether fresh and lovely.

As with her earlier work, the physical world is a tangible presence throughout. Dunmore's love for the sea, coastal landscapes and local flora are all in evidence. Images of natural beauty scattered across the collection lodge in the reader's mind. Although interior spaces feature in some poems, there is always a strong connection to the world beyond. It is as if she is nudging the reader to appreciate that the physical confines forced on us by illness cannot block out the beauty of the physical world or indeed of the world of the imagination. The nature of light and darkness is considered and lamplighters – custodians of the space between light and darkness – appear in several poems. Dunmore creates a sense that, even with all that cannot be known, there will be ways to navigate through the darkness. She acknowledges pain, fear and vulnerability while building a calm acceptance of death as a natural and inevitable part of life. The complexity of the feelings experienced as death approaches is never downplayed. A definite and all-too-human sense of foreboding is palpable and yet there is also comfort, reassurance and even optimism. When Dunmore compares death to a mother's loving embrace in the very last poem, written just ten days before her own death, no reader could fail to be consoled. She is assuring us that death should not be feared, echoing Seamus Heaney's famous last written words: *Noli timere* or "Don't be afraid".

Unsurprisingly, serious illness can make human beings solipsistic, and so poetry about cancer and death is often acutely self-absorbed. One of the most refreshing aspects of *Inside the Wave* is the total absence of this trait. It sets this work apart and is yet another reason why this collection is really special. The harsh personal realities of dealing with serious illness and the dying process are carefully addressed in short bursts that are all the more effective for being so brief. Dunmore's eye is always focused on human connectedness and the shared experience of living and dying. Her feminist sensibility and attentiveness to the world around her are among the most attractive aspects of her writing. A keen awareness of how ordinary lives are impinged upon by political and social upheaval, and her consciousness of the need for constant vigilance around children, add gravitas and another layer of meaning to *Inside the Wave*.

Dunmore explicitly positions herself as belonging to a community of the suffering that includes the terminally ill but also extends well beyond. She has space in her heart and her mind for those enduring oppression and dying in horrific and inhuman circumstances. Her respect for the community of "ordinary souls," and her consciousness of the beauty to be found in ordinary lives which quickly fade from history are subtly conveyed. There are wonderful biographical poems about her father and mother, her children, and the childhood memories that resurfaced during her dying time. We travel with the poet as she gazes backward, seeking a greater understanding of the ebb and flow of individual lives. She imbues these poems with a quality of universality to which the reader can easily relate.

Inside the Wave features in the wonderful retrospective book *Counting Backwards: Poems 1975 – 2017*, published by Bloodaxe. In it, Dunmore's poems from over four decades were brought together at last. There can be no mistaking the female voice at the heart of her work. *Inside the Wave* celebrates female experience in subtle brush strokes and contains striking images that only a female poet would choose. Her poetry skilfully expresses the female perspective in poems that deal with human vulnerability, fear, loss and sadness. In particular, the nurturing nature of motherhood, with its joys and tensions, is like a refrain that plays out across the collection. Furthermore, her poetry is female in its power, honesty, generosity and wisdom. Dunmore's wonderfully brave poems about serious illness and the dying process are also joyous. You won't find better company if you are living in the shadow of death, struggling to come to terms with life's transience, and seeking to make peace with existential questions.

HELEN DUNMORE

My life's stem was cut

My life's stem was cut,
But quickly, lovingly
I was lifted up,
I heard the rush of the tap
And I was set in water
In the blue vase, beautiful
In lip and curve,
And here I am
Opening one petal
As the tea cools.
I wait while the sun moves
And the bees finish their dancing,
I know I am dying
But why not keep flowering
As long as I can
From my cut stem?

My people

My people are the dying,
I am of their company
And they are mine,
We wake in the wan hour
Between three and four,
Listen to the rain
And consider our painkillers.
I lie here in the warm
With four pillows, a light
And the comfort of my phone
On which I sometimes compose,
And the words come easily
Bubbling like notes
From a bird that thinks it is dawn.

My people are the dying.
I reach out to them,
A company of suffering.
One falls by the roadside
And a boot stamps on him,
One lies in her cell, alone,
Without tenderness
Brutally handled
Towards her execution.
I can do nothing.
This is my vigil: the lit candle,
The pain, the breath of my people
Drawn in pain.

The Bridge (1997)

Marin Sorescu

(*Romanian Poet 1936–1996*)

Sorkin, Adam J. & Vianu, Lidia

(*Translators*)

Thrilling moments arose with the discovery of remarkable poets whose names in many cases were familiar but whose work I had never read. A high point was discovering Marin Sorescu. His collection *The Bridge* was written in just five weeks as he was dying from liver cancer. It is authentic and masterful but also a harrowing testament to the experience of dying. There is no pretence and no attempt to hide from or dilute horrifying realities. The struggle to deal with pain, terror, despair and dread has rarely been so impressively articulated. It is not surprising to learn that *The Bridge* inspired a libretto by the American composer Michael Hersch, who had been searching for material that encapsulated his own bitter cancer experience.

A prolific poet and playwright, Marin Sorescu was a giant of 20th-century literature, beloved by Romanian people and highly respected by the literary community across Europe. He arrived on the scene just as a major revival of Romanian poetry was beginning. His body of work was widely translated and published to critical acclaim, ensuring an appreciative audience internationally. Despite living under Ceausescu's tyrannical regime, he was allowed to travel to receive awards and give readings. He managed to build strong literary connections, not least here in Ireland where he was held in high regard by Irish poets including Seamus Heaney and Paul Muldoon. In 1996, the year of his death, he was a nominee for the Nobel Prize in Literature. Although life was extremely restricted under Ceausescu, Sorescu managed to thrive artistically. Like his compatriot poets, he turned to fable and allegory to circumvent state control, mask real intention in his work and maintain his artistic integrity. His satirical poetry and his plays were heavily censored but in general his writing was tolerated. The absurdist, comical, fantastical and playful characteristics of his poetry are remarkably appealing. However, there is no mistaking the underlying seriousness of his work nor his melancholic view of the human condition. Nowhere are these characteristics more evident than in *The Bridge*.

In 1996, on a daily basis from November 1st until the day before his death on December 8th, Sorescu found the strength and courage to write seventy-three of the seventy-five exceptional poems that make up this collection. Initially, his poems were hand-written in an old appointments diary and then read out to his wife, typed and revised. Later, poems were dictated to her and re-drafted verbally. The re-drafting process was rigorous, reflecting Sorescu's determination to deliver on his artistic vision. For instance, the title poem, 'The Bridge', was written on November 2nd and revised on the day before he died, when he introduced the deceptively simple but profoundly moving line "I've never been so scared." In addition, some bleak verse was omitted from the final work at his request. The resultant collection is extraordinary. Themes, images and meaning emerge and then develop. A skilled dramatist, Sorescu creates an inescapable momentum that drives the reader on from one poem to the next, knowing all the while that death is the inevitable end point. His translators beautifully capture this aspect of the work when they refer to it as "a dance of death arranged as a procession of still living poems".

The poems appear in a chronological sequence but there is no mistaking the masterful way in which Sorescu planned the final structure of the collection. *The Bridge* begins with a poem set in daytime, with the poet as the self-aware victim begging God and friends to gather round as he struggles to come to terms with his fate. The collection reaches its climax in the penultimate poem which is anchored in night-time, in isolation, and in the terrible reality of facing imminent death alone. The anguish depicted in the very last poem, written on the eve of his death, hits like a forceful blow. It is no less powerful for being expected. And yet, this final poem, with its veiled reference to the Greek myth of Odysseus and his faithful dog, Argos, subtly suggests a homecoming at the end of a long and difficult journey. It is a reminder that a more complex truth lies beneath what appears at first glance to be straight-forward and plain-speaking poetry. The ambiguity which was a feature of Sorescu's work continued to work its magic in *The Bridge*.

The early poems introduce themes, images, and symbols that Sorescu uses to convey human vulnerability, human frailty and an ever-present sense of growing threat. The theme of a precarious journey with bridges, ladders and ropes to be navigated is introduced early and recurs throughout. It leads to extraordinary images of the poet stumbling, tottering, falling, and even flying, as he moves relentlessly towards death. The frightening loss of control, the feeling of being overwhelmed, and the consequent distress experienced during serious illness, are flawlessly captured in such images. Characters and creatures from Greek mythology appear, reinforcing a message about the universal and timeless nature of the experience of dying. With references to his forerunners, ancestors and even the authors he admired, Sorescu reminds the reader of the fleeting nature of life and the inescapable fate that awaits us all. We see a man in pain, torment and despair who cries out to a God in whom he still believes. In the latter section the poems shorten, the language becomes noticeably dense and spare, and the poems read more and more like prayer. It is intensely personal, searingly honest and heart-breaking.

It is not all doom and gloom, however. Sorescu gives the reader exquisite glimpses of the breath-taking beauty of the natural world and shares moments of brief joy in merely being alive. His characteristic use of a paradoxical punchline at the end of a poem crops up regularly and to great effect. His comic genius and self-deprecating, ironic tone have not deserted him although the humour is understandably of the blackest hue. There is no finer example than the poem 'The Cowardly Coffin', in which Sorescu imagines his own funeral being disrupted by a coffin which refuses to be buried. This bizarre and very funny farce has, of course, a serious undercurrent. There is always welcome relief from tension and anguish when he shows his playful, fanciful, absurdist and richly imaginative side.

Sorescu's style is accessible, his approach direct, and his language appears casual and commonplace at first glance. And yet he shows wonderful artistry and creativity not only in individual poems but also in how this collection is so carefully constructed. In dedicating it "To all who suffer", Sorescu makes clear his intention and his deep sense of solidarity with fellow human beings. He is writing for the community of suffering to which he belongs. In giving voice to that community, he is imploring us to have the courage to look deeply into the horrors of illness and impending death. Consolation can be found not only in the honesty and perceptiveness that shines like a beacon in all these poems, but also in the richness of his poetic voice and the dignity that informs it.

MARIN SORESCU

The Bridge

I balance on something very frail,
A sort of precarious bridge
Blasted apart by the spasms
Of a fierce whirlwind.
A bridge between nothing and nothing,
Which I have not asked to cross.

I've never made
Such grotesque gestures,
Mimicking prayer, defiance, despair …
I'm hurled high in the sky
Among the thunderclaps,
I plummet here below,
Again I'm hurled above.
I've never been so scared.

'Get down from that
Imaginary line.
Don't you understand? It's all over.'
I'm tossed up yet again, slammed back to the ground,
My head whacked against the walls;
I totter, catch hold,
Barely stand on my own.
'I didn't know life
Was an imaginary line,' I say.
This buffeting makes sport with me
On the flimsy plank between earth and sky.

THE BREATH OF CONSOLATION

How far behind I've left the cradle,
Built of the same wood as the bridge,
In which my mother, singing and weeping,
Taught me the cosmic rhythm
I'm in the throes of losing now:
Hush-a-bye! Sleep tight!
'Why didn't you ever tell me that life
Was an imaginary line,
Mother?'

The Cowardly Coffin

It let itself be laid carefully in the grave
By skilled, brawny men
Inured to this.
('Hold it there! A bit more to the right!
That's it, OK! Let go! No, no, not all the way.')

When I finally touched bottom in the grave
(It had to be widened, since they dug it rather narrow),
The coffin gave a quick shudder,
A start,
And shot high above
Dragging the gravediggers along,
Caught in the straps.

The procession was astounded.
What material could the coffin be made of?
Or was there something horrifying
At the bottom of the grave?
The newspapermen required a clarification
And blamed the upcoming elections.

The coffin, which appeared quite ordinary,
Rough-planed planks nailed with 10-penny nails,
Knocked over several crosses,
Banged into the church steeple,
Swung about through the air
(The gravediggers climbed down from trees,
A plum or two in their mouths),
And after a while returned,

THE BREATH OF CONSOLATION

Contrite, to the rim of the grave.
It waited for flowers to be thrown,
And fresh earth.

The women, beginning to weep all over again,
Filed by it.
'Let's get with it, man! Give it another try!
Play out some more rope,
And you, you hold it down.
Two of you men, sit on its lid
To make it heavier.
Others of you, jump on when it touches the ground,
As counterbalance.'

A little this way, a little that way, very carefully,
It descended like lead to the other world.
Then a sudden tremor –
And with a sort of stifled moan,
The narrow end first, as if from a launching pad,
Aerodynamic, it blasted off again.

As late as nightfall, with all manner of tricks,
It would not be buried.
Now it's flying crazily in the sky,
Soon to be shot down
By some rocket or another
From our missile defence.

Say Yes Quickly: A Cancer Tapestry (1997)

Mary Bradish O'Connor

(American writer 1942–2000)

When my capacity to read cancer memoirs buckled under chemotherapy, I retreated to treasured novels and cancer poetry to save my sanity. Luckily, over the preceding months I had accumulated a stockpile of poetry collections and anthologies. Scattered amongst the famous writers were many neglected and unknown poets. In addition, quite a few anthologies included poems by cancer patients publishing for the very first time. I was struck by the vibrancy of some of this work. In confronting the realities of living and dying with cancer, profound experiences were sometimes articulated not only with insight and truth but also with originality, technical skill and poetic style. Biographical information was sketchy and critical reviews often non-existent, so developing a fully rounded picture of many of these works was challenging. Nevertheless, I approached every single collection in hope and expectation. During long months in the infusion chair, one female poet made a profound impact on me and claimed a place in this work by absolute right.

Say Yes Quickly is one of just two published poetry collections by Mary Bradish O'Connor. She chronicles personal struggles that are all too familiar to those of us living with terminal cancer. O'Connor writes about coming to terms with the initial diagnosis, enduring treatment and facing cancer recurrence. The search for acceptance, inner peace and a way to live fully whilst enduring physical, emotional and spiritual suffering is courageously and honestly explored. Throughout this richly layered collection of lyrical poems O'Connor's voice is natural and unforced but also acutely perceptive. The reader is drawn back time and again as the poet gives shape to lived experiences and felt emotions. This is compelling poetry that triggers a strong and empathetic response from the reader.

Fifty-two poems are interspersed with six short prose pieces and eight tankas (short verses). Taken together, they form an intimate chronicle of the poet's thoughts and feelings about her experiences. One of the many joys of *Say Yes Quickly* is O'Connor's skilful use of a mix of poetic forms and her ability to move smoothly and effortlessly between them. Long single stanzas help to convey the inescapable and unyielding reality of cancer and the tsunami of conflicting emotions it generates. The technique of variable line lengths is adopted in many poems to great effect. Short lines – sometimes as short as a word or two – appear frequently, giving the reader a little time to pause, catch their breath and consider. And yet the strong impetus in these stanzas is always to read on, as unexpected twists and turns in mood and emotion are navigated. Some poems begin but also end in wretched moments of fear and dread, but in between there are brief glimpses of the joys of ordinary life. O'Connor turns more and more frequently to the sonnet form as the collection unfolds. In a short prose piece, the poet herself explains:

> The regular format of the structure comforts me …The sonnet's structure acts like a container for my wild, out-of-control emotions of fear, rage, and bitterness. It manages the chaos of cancer's intense feelings and helps me rise above banality when I describe them.

The concluding couplets of many of her sonnets are simply wonderful, conveying the essence of her emotional responses and the hard-won insights gained. Many linger in the mind, with the best taking root. The reader senses O'Connor's commitment to her craft and her careful attention to a rigorous editing process to perfect her work.

O'Connor's versatility is reflected in how she brings the reader up close to pivotal moments in her life in some poems whilst in others she purposefully takes the focus out, exploring the wider world around her and the life that still exists beyond cancer. We are with her in a café with two friends as the invisibility of the grief of her infertility separates her from them, for a time at least. We are with her in the doctor's lounge as she receives her diagnosis. We are with her at the ocean's edge as she struggles to comprehend her utterly changed reality, the isolating nature of cancer, and her sense of immortality forever breached. Poem after poem drives home hard, unvarnished truths about the impact of treatment and the dread that takes hold whilst awaiting results from blood tests and CAT scans. Her poetry is suffused with images of wild storms, howling winds, heavy rain, fog, chilling cold and threatening darkness. A sense of the fragility of life and the ever-present threat of a catastrophe waiting to strike is palpable. Images of cancer as a snake, a dragon and fire, ready to topple, trap or consume catch the intensity of her experiences.

Thankfully, there is also joy and comfort to be found and the book is very much grounded in her sense of place and love for the natural world. She is alive to the transcendent power of nature and celebrates it at every turn, recognising how it sustains her. The landscape of Northern California comes to life as she presents images of seascapes, mountains, glaciers, canyons and creeks. The trees of Northern California –glorious redwoods, cypresses, cottonwoods and oaks – populate her poems together with indigenous wildlife, sea life and birds. The symbolism of birds and animals such as the raven, the hummingbird and the coyote is shrewdly and effectively utilised. There is a vivid rendering of the restorative power of nature for wounded and suffering human beings in many poems. But while she acknowledges its power, O'Connor also hints at nature's fragility. In one poem she references the environmental damage wrought by humans which in turn wreaks havoc on humanity.

Her study of human relationships at a time of crisis is nuanced and delicately done. Over several poems, she honours a loving and caring partner with words that are tender, loving and warm. Yet, she doesn't shy away from reminding us that the dying journey must be taken alone. The complexity of family relationships is alluded to, most poignantly in 'Love Builds a Bridge' which ends with the heart-breaking line:

> Another sweet and sour irony:
> Cancer brought my brother back to me.

The crucial importance of friendship is woven through the collection and celebrated in *Kindred Spirit*. She pays homage to the friends who have carried her through, comparing their support of her to how whales tenderly protect an injured member of their pod. Never shying away from painful realities,

O'Connor expresses her anger and disappointment with someone who failed her by disappearing at the toughest moment of her life. In 'Just Say It' she captures this awful reality for many struggling with cancer. O'Connor succeeds in expressing the highs and lows of complicated human relationships at a time of terminal illness with subtlety and deceptive simplicity.

Tantalising glimpses of the poet appear in her work and suggest a generous, open and quietly attentive nature. Her spirituality is apparent throughout. Belief in God and respect for different spiritual practices including Buddhism and Indigenous American beliefs is tangible. The importance of literature is touched on in one of the short prose pieces. Her innate social and political awareness and concern for the world around her shine. She references the horrors of the war in Bosnia and the racism, sexism and bigotry poisoning American society. In 'The Heartland of America' she foreshadows current events when she acknowledges how white people fail to admit – or indeed even to see – how deeply ingrained racism and bigotry can be in themselves and not just in wider society. All told, the reader finds a poet who is engaged with the world and alive to the sweetness of life but also to its darker and more brutal realities. In the latter half of the collection, the reader senses that O'Connor is coming to terms with her imminent death and finding a way to make fear and uncertainty manageable. Her determination to live with grace, cherishing every moment on what she calls her "dying journey", is surely something many struggling with cancer aspire to

O'Connor was deeply concerned with memory and legacy. Conscious that she had no children to whom she could entrust her memories, she writes in her introduction:

> Cancer prompts me to create my own memory board ... Yes or no?
> I say yes quickly and conjure this: amber beads on a redwood slab, impressions carved into the heartwood, shard of memory left in the clearing for a stranger to find.

That shard of memory has been found, her presence is felt, and she is not forgotten. By including *Say Yes Quickly* in this collection I hope that a wider audience will discover O'Connor's ability to convert cancer's toughest experiences into meaningful, accessible and ultimately consoling poetry. I wish I had known her in life but, as I re-read her poetry, I like to believe that she is drawing breath again and so living on in her work.

Midnight Cancer

is a bottomless pit
where voices echo
around and around
endlessly
repeating the same
prayer:
oh
God
why
me?
Sooner or later, midnight
cancer changes to
morning cancer,
brighter,
more hopeful.
Somewhere the sun
rises warm and round.
Birds are singing.
After a while,
morning cancer melts
into afternoon cancer
where it hides among chores:
cut the grass
clean the downspouts
drain the noodles.
Later, the house falls silent
and even the dog is asleep.
There might or might not be rain.

Without a sound
you are falling,
arms wide and circling.
It's midnight.
You have cancer.

Venerable Bede in Caspar

I

The hummingbird shoots indoors
whirls around
almost at once begins to beat
her wings her whole self
against the skylight, dropping
tiny drops of fear
buzzing and whirring
frantic cheeping
as the brilliant sunshine pours
through the glass.
Long beak half open,
her emerald green body
rests briefly on the ledge
that supports the glass
and now her.
Small clear drops fall continuously
from her body to the ground
where they are lost.
Cat remains on full alert
while I extend the broom
bristles askew
as far as I can.

II

Every three weeks I went in
for a chemo fill-up.
Going where I was told
trying not to be sick

THE BREATH OF CONSOLATION

needles mapping my dropping bloodcount
I napped the intervening weeks
away. Through the windows I watched
winter blow the redwoods
back and forth back and forth.

Come on Sweetie. I won't
hurt you. Grab on
and you can ride out
back to your world.
Rest on this and your terror
will be over. Rest on this
for the trip home.
Throw yourself into this
unexpected predicament.
Turn away from the sun
and such desperate hope.

III
Instantaneous choices
of yes, no
hold on let go.
I give up.
After losing my uterus
after losing my ovaries
after losing my appendix
after losing my omentum
after losing my

immortality my
independence
how do I get out of here?

Flash! She's on it!
Then the truth of the short ride
then the instant of flight
green streak of light straight
to the apple tree straight
into blue freedom.

Say Yes Quickly

Get over it. There's a tear in the fabric
of forever and it's just the way
it is. God didn't tap you on the back
because you were a bad girl and today
you pay for it. You did nothing wrong.
It wasn't all the walks you didn't take
or Irish luck that tossed you headlong
into cancer. Consider this a wake-
up call and live your gift of days with joy.
Walk the edge where air is thin and clear,
where fear can take you further. It's just
another country. Chin up. Step through the door.

Each breath in a miracle.
Each breath out a letting go.

Getting Stronger Every Day

Morning
A thousand years ago
someone's hands arranged these rocks
into walls. I bend
in the doorway, enter
a small dark room –
so this is how it was,
wet earthen smells rising
from the ground, voices
distant and indistinct.
People were busy here,
cool in the noon sun,
warm in the cooling evening.
Outside in the rubbish heaps
tiny painted shards
remember water jugs
and the hands that shaped
the coils.
We struggle to reassemble,
to find the reasoned
structure
in the stones.

Twilight
In the arroyo the ruins stand
simply against a rain-filled sky.
Low walls meet at the join,
Rising gradually upward.
A raven is walking among the rubble.

THE BREATH OF CONSOLATION

I am here at the kiva,
witness to the fallen stones.
Deep in the canyon
we live the beauty of the chaos
until darkness
is complete.

Two A.M.
Coyote yips and howls
from within sandstone shadows.
I am called from my dreams
to a restless campground
and in a flash I understand
how to hold this cancer
I have taken on the road:
not rummaging in rubbish heaps
for shards of meaning
or walking among the ruins
of yesterday's structures,
but holding this moment
against time's broader horizon
and breathing
a grateful blessing.
Outside there is no moon
and no water.
Still, the Trickster sings.
Still, my wild heart beats.

Without: Poems (1998)

Donald Hall

(*American writer 1928–2018*)

Poetry is first among equals when it comes to cancer literature. It is so condensed and so transcendent. There is no finer example of its power and effectiveness than *Without*. This eighty-one-page poetry collection is a brilliant though heartbreaking read and, quite simply, a tour de force. With technical mastery, clarity and precision Hall details the illness and death from leukaemia of his beloved wife, the poet Jane Kenyon. Hall laments for Jane but also celebrates and pays tribute to her life, ensuring that her vivid presence is at the very heart of this work. Beautifully observed recollections of their happy and productive lives reveal their mutual love. Although Jane is the focus and comes alive on the page, Hall weaves in his own struggles to endure suffering and crushing loss and his desperate attempts to transcend grief. *Without* ends with Hall on the path to acceptance and recovery whilst still acknowledging the insidious nature of grief. It is a grief that remained with him to the end of his long life. He never ceased mourning her. Hall stated that he wrote this collection out of absolute necessity following Jane's death but knew that his words would also help others experiencing illness, loss and grief. He was right. There is profound understanding and wonderful companionship to be found in the pages of *Without*.

Donald Hall is a giant of American literature and was the Poet Laureate of the United States from 2006 to 2007. He found success early, built on that success and sustained it over a long and prolific career. Although the greatest acclaim was reserved for his multi-award-winning poetry, his writing in a wide range of other genres, including memoir, literary criticism, academic textbooks, sports journalism, essays, plays, short stories and children's literature, was also esteemed. He first made his editorial mark as the poetry editor of *the Paris Review* and continued to demonstrate his literary editorial skills, not least in the numerous and well-regarded anthologies that bear his stamp. A graduate of Harvard and Oxford universities, Hall wrote his college thesis on W.B. Yeats and shared with the Irish poet a belief in the importance of rigorous revision in the quest for perfection. A distinguished academic career followed and he proved to be a popular and able professor of literature. He developed a strong international presence among both his academic and his literary peers. When he eventually left the academic world, he supplemented his income by working as a literary scout for the publisher Harper & Row and was an active participant on the literary circuit, giving public readings over many years. His successful performance style at public readings, a flavour of which can be found on YouTube, was heavily influenced by the poet Dylan Thomas, whom he met during his Oxford years. Published widely in literary magazines including the *Times Literary Supplement* he developed a wide and devoted public readership over his lifetime.

Following the failure of his first marriage and whilst still teaching in the University of Michigan, 41-year-old Hall met and fell in love with the 22-year-old student poet Jane Kenyon. After three years of marriage and at Jane's insistence, he chose to leave the security of tenured academic life to move permanently to New Hampshire and Eagle Pond, a farm that was in his family for more than a century. The change in environment proved crucial to his continuing development as a writer and transformed his poetry. Embracing their new home, Kenyon and Hall both flourished in their poetic work and in their private lives. Eagle Pond farm became a popular destination for many writers and poets who admired not only Hall's work but also Kenyon's, whose reputation was growing and whose career was blossoming. *Without* gives glimpses of those happy, intimate years together, which were not marred by Jane's bouts of depression and were only seriously shaken when Hall was diagnosed with colon cancer in 1989. With remission and a slow recovery, their idyllic life was briefly restored. Until, that is, Jane was diagnosed with leukaemia in 1994 at the age of 47. The fifteen horrific months that followed and the shock and grief that engulfed Hall are captured in two poetry collections, *Without* (1998) and *The Painted Bed* (2002), and in a tender memoir, *The Best Day the Worst Day: Life with Jane Kenyon* (2005). There is so much to admire in all three works. They share an emotional intensity that speaks powerfully about love, loss and grief. Yet it is the first collection, *Without*, that, for this reader at least, shines the brightest and elicits the deepest response.

What is immediately striking is the brilliance of its structure. The title poem is pivotal, placed at both the physical centre and the creative heart of the collection. It somehow holds all the emotions and experiences that precede and follow Jane's death together. Different from every other poem in the series, it is written in a cathartic and rhetorical style, devoid of punctuation. It marks the awful reality Hall faced. A world without his beloved Jane is a world without colour, without flavour, without season, without meaning, steeped in uncontrollable grief. And yet it is also a world in which Hall still manages to feel an inkling of hope. In this one poem Hall gives an astonishing summation of the overwhelming and suffocating nature of heartbreak and pain. It is interesting to note that this poem was written six months into Jane's treatment and received her approval. Clearly, their shared passion for poetry was a fundamental element of the bond between these two writers.

The first half of the collection chronicles the descent into darkness over fifteen months of illness and ends with Jane's death. The first poem, 'Her Long Illness', is a triumph. It is told at intervals and is interspersed with other poems that replicate and reinforce the central themes. We are brought straight into the unfolding horror of cancer and it seizes our full attention. Chemotherapy, mounting physical and mental side effects, ever increasing suffering, the terrors of bone marrow transplantation and, finally, tentative signs of recovery, are frankly portrayed. The profound emotions generated in both patient and carer are exposed. Love, dread, desperation, rage, fear of death, fear of separation, suicidal thoughts and glimmers of hope all clamour for consideration. Death is ever-present and Hall revives memories of his mother, Lucy, and Jane's mother, Polly, both of whom died during Jane's illness. Two tender and moving elegiac poems capture the essence of both women and honour them. The last poem in the first section, 'Last Days', details over eleven pages the devastating return of leukaemia and the intimate moments shared up to the very point of Jane's death. It reveals how the couple prepared for her death together, working on Jane's last poetry collection, picking hymns for her funeral, writing her obituary and selecting clothes for burial. Friends and loved ones visit while Hall continues to provide for Jane's every physical need as her health disintegrates. They reminisce about travels taken but find deepest comfort in recalling the ordinary routines of their lives that brought daily joy.

Following the title poem, Hall traces the tortuous journey back into the light over the course of one year, and his struggle to find a way to live with grief and despair. In a series of poems shaped as letters addressed to Jane, he gradually replaces the landscape of leukaemia, presented so powerfully in the first half of the collection, with the natural landscape of Eagle Pond farm, their physical and spiritual home. Conversational in tone, these poems mirror the natural desire to bring his beloved wife back to life. In fact, as Hall himself pointed out many years later, this work was slowly bringing his poetic language back to life and writing it became an act of self-healing. The poems are filled with news of family, friends and visits to her grave with the family dog, Gus, and Hall marks all those difficult "firsts" so familiar to the bereaved: the arrival of each new season, Christmas, New Year, the first anniversary of a death.

Permeating the whole collection is Jane's presence, brought vividly to life through Hall's words. He carefully builds up a picture of a woman of courage, wit and humour, living an ordinary life and busy with everyday routines: shopping, walking the dog, baking and gardening. We are also presented with images of a deeply contented woman at work on her poetry and at home in the New Hampshire landscape. The collection ends with a nature poem which Hall himself declared to be heavily influenced by Jane's style. Right to the very end he is consciously and very deliberately celebrating the woman he loved. It is a wonderful poem to bring the collection to a close, displaying a growing awareness of how the cycle of life continues. Hall is moving towards acceptance, emerging from grief and finding a way to endure, to reconnect and begin to move forward with his life and his work.

This remarkable book is a powerful evocation of the cancer experience and the terrible loss and grief it brings. The agony of watching helplessly as a loved one suffers and the shared dread of separation is vividly portrayed. The voice of the carer rings out with courage and poignancy. However, it is Jane's luminous presence which stands at its emotional core. *Without* is a towering achievement and a richly rewarding, although heartrending read.

DONALD HALL

The Ship Pounding

Each morning I made my way
among gangways, elevators,
and nurses' pods to Jane's room
to interrogate the grave helpers
who tended her through the night
while the ship's massive engines
kept its propellers turning.
Week after week, I sat by her bed
with black coffee and the *Globe*.
The passengers on this voyage
wore masks or cannulae
or dangled devices that dripped
chemicals into their wrists.
I believed that the ship
traveled to a harbor
of breakfast, work, and love.
I wrote: "When the infusions
are infused entirely, bone
marrow restored and lymphoblasts
remitted, I will take my wife,
bald as Michael Jordan,
back to our dog and day." Today,
months later at home, these
words turned up on my desk
as I listened in case Jane called
for help, or spoke in delirium,
ready to make the agitated
drive to Emergency again

THE BREATH OF CONSOLATION

for readmission to the huge
vessel that heaves water month
after month, without leaving
port, without moving a knot,
without arrival or destination,
its great engines pounding.

Without

we lived in a small island stone nation
without color under gray clouds and wind
distant the unlimited ocean acute
lymphoblastic leukemia without seagulls
or palm trees without vegetation
or animal life only barnacles and lead
colored moss that darkened when months did

hours days weeks months weeks days hours
the year endured without punctuation
february without ice winter sleet
snow melted recovered but nothing
without thaw although cold streams hurtled
no snowdrop or crocus rose no yellow
no red leaves of maple without october

no spring no summer no autumn no winter
no rain no peony thunder no woodthrush
the book was a thousand pages without commas
without mice oak leaves windstorms
no castles no plazas no flags no parrots
without carnival or the procession of relics
intolerable without brackets or colons

silence without color sound without smell
without apples without pork to rupture gnash
unpunctuated without churches uninterrupted
no orioles ginger noses no opera no

THE BREATH OF CONSOLATION

without fingers daffodils cheekbones
the body was a nation a tribe dug into stone
assaulted white blood broken to shards

provinces invaded bombed shot shelled
artillery sniper fire helicopter gunship
grenade burning murder landmine starvation
the ceasefire lasted forty-eight hours
then a shell exploded in a market
pain vomit neuropathy morphine nightmare
confusion the rack terror the vise

vincristine ara-c cytoxan vp-16
loss of memory loss of language losses
pneumocystis carinii pneumonia bactrim
foamless unmitigated sea without sea
delirium whipmarks of petechiae
multiple blisters of herpes zoster
and how are you doing today I am doing

one afternoon say the sun came out
moss took on greenishness leaves fell
the market opened a loaf of bread a sparrow
a bony dog wandered back sniffing a lath
it might be possible to take up a pencil
unwritten stanzas taken up and touched
beautiful terrible sentences unuttered

the sea unrelenting wave of gray the sea
flotsam without islands broken crates
block after block the same house the mall
no cathedral no hobo jungle the same women
and men they longed to drink hayfields no
without dog or semicolon or village square
without monkey or lily without garlic

Weeds and Peonies

Your peonies burst out, white as snow squalls,
with red flecks at their shaggy centers
in your border of prodigies by the porch.
I carry one magnanimous blossom indoors
and float it in a glass bowl, as you used to do.

Ordinary pleasures, contentment recollected,
blow like snow into the abandoned garden,
overcoming the daisies. Your blue coat
vanishes down Pond Road into imagined snowflakes
with Gus at your side, his great tail swinging,

but you will not reappear, tired and satisfied,
and grief's repeated particles suffuse the air –
like the dog yipping through the entire night,
or the cat stretching awake, then curling
as if to dream of her mother's milky nipples.

A raccoon dislodged a geranium from its pot.
Flowers, roots, and dirt lay upended
in the back garden where lilies begin
their daily excursions above stone walls
in the season of old roses. I pace beside weeds

and snowy peonies, staring at Mount Kearsarge
where you climbed wearing purple hiking boots.
"Hurry back. Be careful, climbing down."
Your peonies lean their vast heads westward
as if they might topple. Some topple.

Of Mutability (2010)

Jo Shapcott
(*English writer. Born 1953*)

Jo Shapcott's *Of Mutability* perfectly exemplifies the force of poetry, most especially for those living and dying with cancer. This slim volume contains just forty-five poems, the vast majority of which are shorter than a page in length. It may be modest in physical scale but it has a depth, complexity and sophistication that is more than equal to the task of probing how the cancer experience changes forever our sense of the world. The themes of mortality and change dominate in poems that reveal an inventive convergence of fear and hope, seriousness and playfulness, uncertainty and optimism. Surreal wit, warmth and vitality leap from the page together with glorious moments of joy. It is not at all surprising, therefore, to discover that the creator of this engaging and life-affirming work is a much admired and multi-award-winning poet.

London-born Jo Shapcott encountered tragic loss early in her life with the death of her parents when she was aged just eighteen. Despite this life-altering experience, her undergraduate years at Trinity College Dublin were happy ones. Postgraduate study commenced in Oxford and eventually led to a scholarship to Harvard where she studied under Seamus Heaney. Her working life began in arts administration. In 1985, her stature as a poet was established when she won the U.K.'s National Poetry Competition. Three years later, her first poetry collection was published to great acclaim. A flourishing academic career beckoned, and she is currently Professor of Creative Writing at Royal Holloway, University of London. Over the years, her reputation as a critic, an editor and a broadcaster has grown. Diagnosed in 2003 with breast cancer, she went through the all-too-familiar tough treatment cycle but emerged cancer-free and is in long-term remission. Her cancer experience triggered a creative need to interrogate how her sense of the world had changed and led to her first poetry collection in twelve years. *Of Mutability*, published in 2010, promptly won the overall Costa Book of the Year.

The importance of the paratextual is self-evident, for a librarian at least. All the material that surrounds the main text including titles, cover design, formatting and blurbs can play a critical role in attracting the reader. With *Of Mutability*, the paratextual works brilliantly. I was struck by the cleverness of the choice of book title and the layers of meaning it contains. Firstly, mutability is a great word for a book about cancer. It is suggestive of decay, degeneration and death but also of change, transformation and survival. The word has added significance for those of us living with Chronic Lymphocytic Leukaemia, as a mutated form of this blood cancer is associated with slower cancer growth and a better long-term prognosis. Secondly, mutability is a word which evokes literary memories. Many poets have tackled the theme of mutability, most notably Shelley, Shakespeare and Wordsworth. Shapcott is paying homage to that poetic tradition. I first encountered lines from Shelley's poem 'Mutability' in the gothic novel *Frankenstein* written by his wife, Mary Shelley. Consequently, the word is forever linked in my mind with the unsettling reality of how little control we have over our lives. Perpetual change is the only constant. Lastly, Shapcott pays homage to the English sculptor, photographer and installation artist Helen Chadwick whose first major solo exhibition was entitled *Of Mutability*. The poet acknowledges Chadwick as the presiding spirit of this collection, supplying titles as well as inspiration. Shapcott's ear for provocative titles results in some unforgettable ones for this collection including 'Uncertainty Is Not a Good Dog', 'Hairless', 'Tea Death' and 'Somewhat Unravelled'.

Of Mutability has been described by the poet herself as emotionally autobiographical. Although this work is clearly a sequence of meditations on mortality, it is notable that the word cancer never appears, yet the impact of cancer on both mind and body is deftly portrayed. The collection opens with a two-stanza title poem that brings the reader face to face with serious illness. The subtle tonal shifts of this first poem set the tone for the collection as a whole. Dread, fear and uncertainty stalk the first stanza but shift in the second to optimism, learning, life and hope, whilst retaining a strong note of realism. Not only central themes but also key motifs and symbols are introduced in this title poem.

One important motif is the word "cell" which alludes to cancer but also to the nature of the body and the world of science, two subjects close to Shapcott's heart. It is interesting that the word "cell" appears in just two of the early poems and only re-appears again in four of the closing ones. The gravitas of this word is felt all the more because of its judicious placement. The focus in the opening poems is on cells that are in crisis and multiplying rapidly. When we reach the later poems, cells are referred to as fresh and altered. The reader – and perhaps the poet herself – is urged to forget about what is taking place in the author's cells. When we reach the joyful poem 'Procedure', we are told that the chaos that has assailed her cells is a thing of the past and we are invited to share in this ecstatic moment.

In exploring how the relationship with the body changes under the onslaught of cancer and its treatment Shapcott uses the metaphor of water to powerful effect. The physical experiences of liquidity and permeability are depicted, with descriptions of her body as belonging to a watery city in 'La Serenissima', and being a drop of water in 'Deft'. Bubbles, antibubbles, sweat and urine all feature as metaphors. She nails the sense of a physical body mutating, boundaries dissolving and transformation taking place. Pavements ripple underfoot. Traffic swims. There is a surreal quality to her choice of metaphors that fits perfectly the experiences of serious illness, as many who know cancer treatment will attest to.

The pivotal image of looking skyward is introduced in the title poem and is used effectively and creatively throughout, each time providing shifts of viewpoints and meaning. We are challenged to consider how small one human life is in the context of the scale and complexity of the sky above us. We are reminded of how serious illness changes our physical viewpoint, as we spend hours in bed forced to look upward. It also transforms how we see our inner world, opening us up to different ways of considering life and death at a time of crisis. Shapcott uses the image of the sky to nudge the reader into thinking about climate change. The destructive signs of climate change are first referenced in 'Era', when she alludes to changing migratory bird patterns. Later in the collection, in 'St Bride's', the destruction wrought by aerial warfare on a city of innocent people tells readers unfamiliar with Shapcott's work that here is a poet deeply concerned about political matters. Naturally, that acute political awareness is somewhat subjugated at a time when the poet is mired in personal crisis. Nevertheless, direct and oblique references to the Iraq war appear, most impressively when she juxtaposes the invasion of Iraq with that grim personal moment in time when cancer treatment begins. In Shapcott's work, the disarray of the body is matched by the political chaos of a world where the Gulf stream is slowing, ice shelves are collapsing, and mass killing is taking place for spurious reasons that seem as capricious as cancer itself.

It is exhilarating to read such inventive poetry. She introduces a diversity of subjects as she meditates on mutability. Landscape is one. The modern cityscape of London is a living and perpetually changing presence all through the collection. In a short sequence of poems celebrating trees, Shapcott considers how trees record and reflect the changes that take place in their natural environment yet remain seemingly impervious to humans. The mental degeneration of a beloved aunt with Alzheimer's is explored in the touching and gently humorous poem 'Somewhat Unravelled'. A couple mutate together in the poem 'Abishag', where the nature of age, mortality and love are probed.

Shapcott's feminist voice is also an erotic and sensual one, always deeply appreciative of life. In the poem 'Hairless'', for example, she describes the skin on a bald woman's head in her unique and poetic way. Although Shapcott is writing about death and change, unease and dread, uncertainty and loss, there is something truly glorious and life-affirming about *Of Mutability*, which makes it that rarity in literature that readers suffering with cancer long for. Honest, serious, inventive, and playful, it is suffused with a love for life and forever conscious of the possibility of joy even when life itself is under dire threat. In the final analysis, who could resist a collection that ends with the euphoria of survival and a poet poised for a future, changed but unbowed?

Jo Shapcott

Of Mutability

Too many of the best cells in my body
are itching, feeling jagged, turning raw
in this spring chill. It's two thousand and four
and I don't know a soul who doesn't feel small
among the numbers. Razor small.
Look down these days to see your feet
mistrust the pavement and your blood tests
turn the doctor's expression grave.

Look up to catch eclipses, gold leaf, comets,
angels, chandeliers, out of the corner of your eye,
join them if you like, learn astrophysics, or
learn folksong, human sacrifice, mortality,
flying, fishing, sex without touching much.
Don't trouble, though, to head anywhere but the sky.

Hairless

Can the bald lie? The nature of the skin says not:
it's newborn-pale, erection-tender stuff,
every thought visible – pure knowledge,
mind in action – shining through the skull.
I saw a woman, hairless absolute, cleaning.
She mopped the green floor, dusted bookshelves,
all cloth and concentration, Queen of the moon.
You can tell, with the bald, that the air
speaks to them differently, touches their heads
with exquisite expression. As she danced
her laundry dance with the motes, everything
she ever knew skittered under her scalp.
It was clear just from the texture of her head,
she was about to raise her arms to the sky;
I covered my ears as she prepared to sing, to roar.

Jo Shapcott

Stargazer

If I'm not looking at you,
forgive; if I appear
to be scanning the sky,
head thrown back, curious,
ecstatic, shy, strolling
unevenly across the floor
in front of you, my audience,
forgive, and forget what's
happening in my cells.
It's you I'm thinking of
and, voice thrown upwards,
to you I'm speaking, you.

I'm trying to keep this simple
in the time left to me:
luckily, it's a slow
and selective degeneration.
I'm hoping, mainly, to stay present
and straight up despite
the wrong urge that's taken hold,
to say everything, all
at once, to everyone, which
is what I'd like if only
I could stay beyond this moment.

Procedure

This tea, this cup of tea, made of leaves,
made of the leaves of herbs and absolute

almond blossom, this tea, is the interpreter
of almond, liquid touchstone which lets us
scent its true taste at last and with a bump,

in my case, takes me back to the yellow time
of trouble with blood tests, and cellular
madness, and my presence required

on the slab for the surgery, and all that mess
I don't want to comb through here because
it seems, honestly, a trifle now that steam

and scent and strength and steep and infusion
say thank you thank you thank you for the then, and now

Every Riven Thing (2010)

Christian Wiman

(American writer. Born 1966)

Christian Wiman is one of only two writers whose work appears twice in this collection. *Every Riven Thing*, like his memoir, *My Bright Abyss*, delves into the poet's personal experiences and tackles the timeless questions many readers living with cancer grapple with. It is thrilling to discover poetry that connects the reader so intensely with the realities of the struggle with cancer, suffering and grief but also with the presence of faith. Wiman explores these themes with subtlety and intricacy, using a poetic language that is simply stunning. *Every Riven Thing* is filled with compelling poetry; concentrated, serious and full of lament but also playful and even humorous at times. It is imbued with love for life and for the moments of joy that are as much a part of human existence as suffering.

It is useful for the reader to know something of Wiman's personal journey as a means of understanding his work more fully. Born in West Texas, he was raised in a fundamentalist religious tradition and in a culture steeped in the gun violence which is so alien to European sensibilities. From his college years on, he distanced himself from that culture and from his troubled relationship with his father. He built a successful life as a poet, an essayist, an editor and a translator. In 2003, the career-enhancing opportunity to edit *Poetry* (a world leading poetry journal) at a time when it had received a massive financial bequest proved irresistible. Just as his career was flourishing, however, a series of major events happened in quick succession that fundamentally altered the course of his life. He stopped writing, feeling that poetry had died in him, and struggled to cope with the loss of what had been his life's purpose. He fell in love, married and felt his solitary life opening up towards a shared future. Spontaneously, if hesitantly at first, prayer became a central part of his life with his partner. Less than a year later, at the age of thirty-nine, he was diagnosed with an incurable blood cancer. Wiman found himself returning to the church. As he explained in a 2007 essay:

> ... what extreme grief has given me is the very thing it seemed first to obliterate: a sense of life beyond the moment, a sense of hope. This is not simply a hope for my own life, though I do have that. It is not hope for heaven or any sort of explainable afterlife ... it is hope toward God."[1]

In the midst of these tumultuous experiences, Wiman's desire and ability to write returned. Poetry once again flowed.

Every Riven Thing is his first poetry collection created in the aftermath of the trauma of diagnosis. The sheer quality of Wiman's craft and the magnitude of his talent are everywhere in evidence. They are in the carefully honed language, the quirky lineation, the nod to poetic traditions and the variety of poetic forms used. He draws the reader into his struggles, carefully constructing the collection around three sections, each with a distinct focus. Section one reveals the anguish of his cancer experience. Section two explores the extremes of grief and despair encountered. In the final section Wiman focuses with remarkable intensity and truth on his faith. Permeating the entire work is the search for an understanding of suffering, helplessness, mortality and life itself, and a consciousness of both the presence and the absence of God.

One of the most pleasurable and indeed memorable aspects of *Every Riven Thing* is its strong sense of place. The harsh and barren natural landscape, the dwellings, the backyards, the characters, even the sounds of West Texas are brought lovingly to life, adding local colour to this evocative work. This is evidenced in three standout poems, 'Five Houses Down', 'Sitting Down to Breakfast Alone' and the longest poem, 'The Reservoir'. Read aloud, the musicality of his poetry is striking. The Texan cadences sing out authentically.

---

[1] Wiman essay 'Gazing into the Abyss' in *The American Scholar*, Summer 2007.

It is little surprise therefore to learn that Wiman is passionate about the work of Patrick Kavanagh, a poet renowned for his use of colloquial language.

The honesty of Wiman's poetry is laid bare most movingly in poems about his family. He conveys his deep love for his wife throughout and she is the subject of the final poem 'Gone for the Day, She is the Day'. He chooses to end this poem, and so the collection, with the word 'love'. In a quintessentially Wiman way he is referencing not only human love but also the love of God. The most disturbing personal poem is also the most powerful. 'Not Altogether Gone' is a seven-part, mercilessly honest depiction of his father. Wiman doesn't flinch from portraying the truth of who his father was and the troubled nature of their relationship. Deeply conflicted, the poet also conveys his love for his father and the grief that took hold following his death.

It is the stark description of Wiman's cancer experiences in the first section that sets the tone for the collection as a whole. In 'After the Diagnosis'', The Mole', and 'Darkcharms,' Wiman pulls no punches in his portrayal of the devastating realities of the disease. What immediately follows this explicit focus on illness is an unforgettable title poem. With its language of paradox, its emphasis on the broken nature of living things, and its deeply moving account of how we experience God, in this poem Wiman connects us with the abstract struggles of mortality and of faith. He achieves this with just nine words that feature at the start of each stanza and in a standalone last line. "God goes belonging to every riven thing he's made" is repeated five times. Using punctuation alone, the poet changes the meaning each time. So much is conveyed in just twenty-one carefully metered lines. We are given a sense of a God who belongs to everyone and every thing. He writes of the experience of both God's presence and God's absence. We see how man is riven not just physically but also emotionally and spiritually, and how the objects of earth have a nearness to God that man yearns for but struggles to attain. Immediately following 'Every Riven Thing' is a poem in the form of a prayer. This form then dominates the final section. He addresses God directly, pleading to be heard, compelled to believe but struggling to make sense of his faith in a God of mystery. It is the truest depiction of the human longing for spiritual consolation that I've found in my journey through cancer literature.

Wiman has forged something powerful, original and intense out of personal suffering and grief. His poetic language of faith, particularly strong in the last section, is profound. We are not presented with easy answers. Instead, Wiman interrogates how suffering can move us toward God and a sense of hope. For many years now I have been drawn back to this work and compelled to consider my own struggles with faith. I still cannot claim to fully understand Wiman's poetry, finding meanings difficult to pin down. It hardly matters, though, as I get lost in its honesty, beauty and mystery every time. Most of all, it is his interrogation of the possibility of spiritual consolation that captivates.

CHRISTIAN WIMAN

After the Diagnosis

No remembering now
when the apple sapling was blown
almost out of the ground.
No telling how,
with all the other trees around,
it alone was struck.
It must have been luck,
he thought for years, so close
to the house it grew.
It must have been night.
Change is a thing one sleeps through
when young, and he was young.
If there was a weakness in the earth,
a give he went down on his knees
to find and feel the limits of,
there is no longer.
If there was one random blow from above
the way he's come to know
from years in this place,
the roots were stronger.
Whatever the case,
he has watched this tree survive
wind ripping at his roof for nights
on end, heats and blights
that left little else alive.
No remembering now ...
A day's changes mean all to him
and all days come down
to one clear pane

THE BREATH OF CONSOLATION

through which he sees
among all the other trees
this leaning, clenched, unyielding one
that seems cast
in the form of a blast
that would have killed it,
as if something at the heart of things,
and with the heart of things,
had willed it.

This Mind of Dying

God let me give you now this mind of dying
fevering me back
into consciousness of all I lack
and of that consciousness becoming proud:

> *There are keener griefs than God.*
> *They come quietly, and in plain daylight,*
> *leaving us with nothing, and the means to feel it.*

My God my grief forgive my grief tamed in language
to a fear that I can bear.
Make of my anguish
more than I can make. Lord, hear my prayer.

Every Riven Thing

God goes, belonging to every riven thing he's made
sing his being simply by being
the thing it is:
stone and tree and sky,
man who sees and sings and wonders why

God goes. Belonging, to every riven thing he's made,
means a storm of peace.
Think of the atoms inside the stone.
Think of the man who sits alone
trying to will himself into a stillness where

God goes belonging, To every riven thing he's made
there is given one shade
shaped exactly to the thing itself:
under the tree a darker tree;
under the man the only man to see

God goes belonging to every riven thing. He's made
the things that bring him near,
made the mind that makes him go.
A part of what man knows,
apart from what man knows,

God goes belonging to every riven thing he's made.

Gone for the Day, She is the Day

Dawn is a dog's yawn, space
in bed where a body should be,
a nectared yard, night surviving
in wires through which what voices,
what needs already move – and the mind
nibbling, nibbling at Nothingness
like a mouse at cheese:

Spring!

*

Sometimes one has the sense
that to say the name
God is a great betrayal,
but whether one is betraying
God, language, or one's self
is harder to say.

*

Gone for the day, she is the day
opening in and around me
like flowers she planted in our yard.
Christ. Not flowers.
Gone for the day, she is the day
razoring in with the Serbian roofers,
and ten o'clock tapped exactly
by the one bad wheel of the tortilla cart,

THE BREATH OF CONSOLATION

and the newborn's noonday anguish
eased. And the *om* the mind
makes of traffic and the bite
of reality that brings it back.
And the late afternoon afterlight
in which a much-loved dog lies
like a piece of precocious darkness
lifting his ears at threats, treats, comings, goings …

*

To love is to feel your death
given to you like a sentence,
to meet the judge's eyes
as if there were a judge,
as if he had eyes,
and love.

Still Life (2019)

Ciaran Carson

(*Irish writer 1948–2019*)

I first read Ciaran Carson's poetry whilst studying the politics of Northern Ireland in University College Dublin in the early 1990s. The impact was immediate and intense. *Belfast Confetti* conveyed the truth of the claustrophobic atmosphere of Belfast and the terrible normalisation of dysfunctional and malevolent life during the Troubles far more profoundly than much of the academic work I was ploughing through at that time. Although literature about Northern Ireland is fertile ground for the reader and there are many great books on the subject, it was decades before I encountered two novels that are as original and as insightful as Carson's poetry. Like *Belfast Confetti*, Anna Burns' *Milkman* and Louise Kennedy's *Trespasses* vividly capture grim features of life in Northern Ireland during the Troubles. Burns and Kennedy bring the female perspective to life, adding the horrors of sexual surveillance and coercion to the toxic mix of realities and oppressive tenor previously revealed by Carson. From the moment of discovery on, I looked forward to every new Carson work. Saddened to read of his death from lung cancer in 2019, I expected his last poetry collection to be a triumph but never imagined that it would also prove to be such a perfect fit for this book.

Born on the lower Falls Road in Belfast and educated at Queen's University, Ciaran Carson was a member of the Belfast Group, a workshop of extraordinary writers that met once a week for a decade from the early 1960s and included Seamus Heaney, Paul Muldoon and Bernard MacLaverty. A colossus of the literary world, Carson was a prolific poet who never wrote the same book twice. Every new collection was a departure, often ground-breaking, always inventive and frequently prize-winning. Carson's prose was as varied and adventurous as his poetry and included novels, a memoir and studies of Irish traditional music. The roots of his fascination with language no doubt lie in his childhood years when Irish was spoken at home. He moved from that bilingual beginning into a multilingual world, eventually becoming a polyglot and a renowned translator. Carson's love for the vernacular added yet another layer of richness to his poetic language. Passionate about Irish music, which he both wrote and played, he carried a sense of rhythm and storytelling from that rich tradition into his writing. The visual arts became a lifelong passion and featured prominently in his writing. The breadth and depth of Carson's engagement with the arts was no doubt nourished by his work, first with the Arts Council of Northern Ireland and later as a Professor of Poetry at Queen's University and the Founding Director of the Seamus Heaney Centre for Poetry. Always attentive to the global cultural world, Carson nevertheless remained deeply rooted in his home city of Belfast. In book after book, he draws his readers into its streets and parks, showing us a wounded city that is still full of possibility. The haunting echoes of the destruction and chaos wrought during the years of conflict, a conflict that indelibly marked the city and its people, reverberate in his writing. In true Carson style, he gathered these diverse strands together one final time to create something fresh and original with his last poetry collection.

 Carson's creativity was unleashed by his terminal diagnosis. In just six months and as he underwent chemotherapy, he produced the seventeen ekphrastic poems that make up *Still Life*. At first reading it may seem like a straightforward homage to the power of art. As the punning title suggests, however, *Still Life* has layers of meaning ripe for discovery. A quintessential storyteller, he brings the reader on a journey in each poem and across poems. It is a trip full of surprising twists and turns, anecdotes and echoes, and the most extraordinary connections all woven together with enviable ease. Yet it also works brilliantly if simply taken as a tribute to art. The book is structured around paintings by renowned French, Italian, Flemish, English, Spanish and local artists that range in time from the 16th to the 21st century. Each poem details the poet's response to a painting as he moves through time and memory. Clearly Carson is as much at home in the world of great painting as he is on his beloved Belfast streets. His love of art is informed by research and he references books that proved invaluable. No reader could hope for a more inspiring introduction to art than

Carson's unique collection. (I only wish that he had brought his poetic eye to bear on El Greco's *The Burial of the Count of Orgaz*, a celebrated vision of the immense consolation of faith.) With Carson's eye for detail, teacher's gift for sharing knowledge, and mastery of language, every painting is brought to life in the reader's mind. No doubt many will go in search of Carson's eclectic mix of paintings armed with *Still Life*.

There is so much more than the power of art to discover, however. Stoical in the face of his terminal illness, Carson conveys a sense of both calm resignation and innate curiosity. Anger and despair are nowhere in evidence. Carson references his illness throughout with seemingly casual asides about hospital visits, chemotherapy and radiotherapy treatments. He cautions readers to *never mind the death in the foreground* yet ensures that we are at all times conscious of and attentive to its grave presence. In *Still Life* we discover a poet negotiating his own path through terminal cancer just as he had previously done through the Belfast of The Troubles. We feel we are right by his side on his journey, losing ourselves to find ourselves. Words and images of encircling darkness, shadow, gloom, decay and death are intricately woven into the collection's fabric. The word *cell*, heavy with meaning, is introduced early, reappears, and is also subtly alluded to in other words including "cellar" and "cellophane". He creates an unforgettable image of cancer treatment by referencing Vermeer's famous and much-loved work *The Lacemaker*, in his poem 'Jeffrey Morgan, Hare Bowl, 2008.'

With characteristic inventiveness, Carson explores death not just as a natural part of the cycle of life but also in its sudden, cruel, and arbitrary manifestations. On the micro level, an account is given of an experiment to discover how long it takes a lemon to completely rot. At the macro level, memories resurface of the human cost of devastating bombings of Belfast. The work of an artist deeply affected by a visit to Hiroshima sparks painful memories of Bloody Friday in Belfast in 1972, when a sequence of bombings in a short period of time killed nine people and injured many more. Carson conveys the absolute horror of both events, one through his description of a work of art, the other triggered by a buried personal memory. There is a fearlessness in how Carson chooses to look into the void. Yet, as he takes stock, he knows that imminent death is only one part of a much bigger story. This collection is also suffused with light, with bright colours and with a wealth of reminders of both natural and man-made patterns of regeneration and transformation. Windows recur throughout as Carson interrogates how we perceive the world around us. They frame the ceaseless patterns of regrowth and renewal and open up Carson's world to the world beyond. It is a world brimming with life that is regenerating itself not only in nature, but also in Belfast's built environment, and ultimately in the indomitable human spirit. Carson's wife, Deirdre, is a constant presence. She is at his side on daily walks around Belfast Waterworks Park. She is an integral part of the conversations and meditations, past and present, that bring each artwork alive and open up the richness of Carson's inner life to the reader. An intimate and celebratory tone runs through the collection. It is no accident that the final poem, entitled 'James Allen, *The House with the Palm Trees*, c.1979' brings the collection to a close with a triple declaration of love for the world and for life itself.

Still Life is a tender and profoundly moving testament to everything that Carson cherished, most especially life itself. Although it has commonalities with other poetry collections chosen for this book, it is also unique. The major themes of cancer literature are present. There is a keen sense of approaching death as he navigates cancer treatment and contemplates life in all its complexity and ambiguity. The happiness of married love and the deep well of a lifetime of shared memories are celebrated. A determination to continue to live a fully engaged life, cherishing every precious moment of the remaining time, is palpable. Solace – for poet and reader – is found in the ceaseless regeneration of life so beautifully captured in his words. Complex yet accessible, full of warmth, freshness and inventiveness, it is remarkably life-affirming poetry. What a joy it is to read and share.

Claude Monet,
Artist's Garden at Vétheuil, 1880

Today I thought I'd just take a lie-down, and drift. So here I am
Listening to the tick of my mechanical aortic valve –
        overhearing, rather, the way
It flits in and out of consciousness. It's a wonder what goes on
        below the threshold.
It's quiet up here, just the muted swoosh of the cars on the
        Antrim Road.
And every so often the shrill of a far-off alarm or the squeal
        of brakes;
But yesterday some vandal upended the terracotta pot of
        daffodils
In our little front garden, that's not even as big, when I
        consider it,
As the double bed I'm lying on. Behind the privet hedge,
        besides the daffodils
There's pansies, thyme and rosemary. A Hebe bush. A laurel.
        Ruefully
I scuffed the spilled earth and pebbles with my shoe and
        thought of Poussin –
Was it Poussin? – and his habit of bringing back bits of
        wood, stones,
Moss, lumps of earth from his rambles by the Tiber; and the
        story of him
Reaching among the ruins for a handful of marble and
        porphyry chips
And saying to a tourist, 'Here's ancient Rome.' So, here's
        Glandore Avenue.

THE BREATH OF CONSOLATION

So different now from thirty years ago, the corner shop at
        the interface
Torched and the roadway strewn with broken glass and rubble.

There was something beautiful about the tossed daffodils all
        the same.
I'd never really taken them under my notice these past few
        difficult weeks.
It's late March, some of them beginning to turn and wilt and
        fade, heads
Drooping, papery at the tips, desiccated, or completely gone,
        reduced to calyx.
So many shades of yellow when you look at them. Gorse.
        Lemon. Mustard.
Honey. Saffron. Ochre. But then any word you care to mention
        has so many
Shades of meaning, and the flower itself goes under different
        names.
Narcissus. Daffadowndilly. Lent lily. So we wander down the
        road of what it is
We think we want to say. Etymologies present themselves,
        like daffodil
From asphodel – who knows where the *d* came from? –
        the flower
Of the underworld. They say it grows profusely in the meadows
        of the dead,
Like a buttercup on its branching stem. And I see a galaxy of
        buttercups in

A green field, and the yellow of the tall sunflowers in Monet's
    Garden at Vétheuil
That flank the path where the woman and the two children
    stand commemorated.
Strange how a smear of colour, like a perfume, resurrects
    the memory
Of another, that which I meant to begin with. 'Asphodel, that
    greeny flower.'

I'd just found the book I had in mind – *What Painting Is*
    by James Elkins –
When the vandal struck. *Thud*. What the …? The gate clanged.
    I looked out
The bay window to see a figure scarpering off down the street
    to the interface …
What a book, though. I have it before me, open at this colour
    plate, jotting notes
Into a jotter, which I'll work up later into what you're
    reading now.
'The detail I'm reproducing here is a graveyard of scattered
    brush hairs
And other detritus,' said Elkins. 'At the centre left, glazed over
    by Malachite Green,
Are two crossed brush hairs, one of them bent almost at a
    right angle.
Just below them are two of Monet's own hairs, fallen into the
    wet paint.'
Brushstrokes laid down every which way. Jiggles. Jabs.
    Impulsive

THE BREATH OF CONSOLATION

Twists and turns. Gestures that 'depend on the inner feelings
    of the body,
And the fleeting momentary awareness of what the hand might
    do next.'
You listen to the body talking, exfoliating itself cell after cell.
    I saw it
Happening just now in the dust-motes drifting through this
    ray of sunlight.

So everything gets into the painting, wood-smoke from the
    studio stove,
The high pollen count of a high summer's day *en plein air* by
    the Seine.

The detail is so magnified it is impossible to tell what it is of,
    if you didn't,
Like Elkins, know. The visual field looks like a field. Shades
    of umber, khaki, mud,
And other greens beside the malachite. It could stand for
    anything it seems
In Monet's garden – or *Garden*, rather – as Poussin's handful
    of porphyry
Is Rome and of the days of the fall of Rome. I want it to go to
    the stately tune
Of a Poussin painting, *Landscape with a Man Washing His Feet
    by a Fountain,*
Say, where a woman sweeps by, balancing a basket on her head,
    and an old man

In blue dreams full-length on the grass. There are milestones
    and tombs,
And puddles on the road, and you can just imagine the
    whispering of the cistern.
A line of blue hills in the distance is contoured like a
    monumental sentence.
It's beautiful weather, the 30th of March, and tomorrow the
    clocks go forward.
How strange it is to be lying here listening to whatever it is
    is going on.
The days are getting longer now, however many of them I
    have left.
And the pencil I am writing this with, old as it is, will easily
    outlast their end.

Angela Hackett,
Lemons on a Moorish Plate, 2013

We'd been talking about how back in the day we'd nothing
    much of anything,
Though what there was to wear – the uniform! – was too big.
    The sleeves
Drooped well below the fingertips. It gave you room to grow
    into. Years loomed.
Day after day, summer after summer, days were immeasurably
    longer then,
And the one tin bathful of hot water did the several children
    one after the other.
Then it seemed in no time at all you were into your teens.
    Because your birthday
Fell a week before Christmas – December the 18th – you'd have
    to make do
With the merest token of a family present. A set of bath salts,
    maybe, or a bar
Of lemon soap the simulacrum of a lemon, and we tried
    to remember
If such a thing came wrapped in tissue paper like the fruit
    itself, or was it
See-through cellophane? Then to summon up the names
    of yesteryear –
Yardley's April Violets; Mornay White Heather; Lenthéric
    Tweed! It's the 1960s,
And I see myself wondering what would be appropriate to buy
    for my mother,
Dazzled by the cornucopian Christmas window display of the
    chemist's shop.

All this, believe it or not, was apropos of Angela Hackett's
    painting –
Because when looking at a thing we often drift into a memory
    of something else.
However tenuous the link. Five years and more – ever since I
    bought it
For your birthday – it's been hanging on our bedroom wall,
    pleasing us
To look at it from time to time to see different things in it.
    Only now has it
Occurred to us to talk about or of it at this length, the lemons –
    three of them –
Proceeding in an anticlockwise swirl from pale lemon to a
    darker yellow
To an almost orange, tinged with green – degrees, we speculate,
    of ripeness
Or decay. You know how lemons, if left too long in the bowl,
    one or two from time
To time will show a blush of green, a dimple or a bruise of
    bluish green
That overnight becomes a whitish bloom? So we think Angela
    Hackett's lemons
Might be on the turn. Though it's possible the green tinge
    might be an echo
Of the two limes I haven't mentioned until now, nestled in
    against the lemons
On the indigo-and-white Moorish plate, all of which
    complicates the picture.

THE BREATH OF CONSOLATION

It gave us pause for thought. How long does it take, we
        wondered, for a lemon
To completely rot? We imagined a time-lapse film, weeks
        compressed into
Seconds, the lemon changing hue, developing that powdery
        bloom, then suddenly
Collapsing into itself to leave a shrunken, pea-sized, desiccated
        husk – the flesh
Evaporated, breathed into the atmosphere as it transpires.
        And that is why
On the 26th of March 2019 we set up the lemon experiment.
        On the avocado-and-aubergine-coloured
Moroccan saucer we bought in Paris we set up a fresh lemon and
        a banana whose peel,
We are led to believe, releases ethylene gas and hence ripens
        any other fruit
With which it comes into contact. We wanted to see with
        our own eyes
The end of the life cycle of the lemon. I write this on the
        6th of April. The banana has gone
Black except at the tips. The lemon looks as fresh as ever.
        We've just been for our daily walk
Around the Waterworks. Ducks are kicking up a racket.
        A blackbird sings
From a blackthorn bush. And we enter into Glandore from
        the Antrim Road
How clean and fresh and green are the newly sprung leaves
        of the chestnut tree!

Canaletto,
The Stonemason's Yard, c. *1725*

Here we are again at the waste ground of 1 Hopefield Avenue,
        and behind
The chain-link fencing is a big yellow JCB emblazoned
        McNABNEY BROS
That wasn't there yesterday; where we saw the goldfinch
        two years ago,
Perched feeding on a thistle-head. Weeds have been culled,
        rubble levelled,
Trenches dug in preparation for whatever. An apartment block?
        If so, for how much
Longer will the gable wall of No. 3 be visible? It had passages
        of inexplicable brickwork
We liked to try to make something of, to say nothing of the
        ghost of the chimney flue of No. 1 –

The kind of thing that had I been a painter I'd have liked to put
        into a painting –
I can see a landscape by Tony Swain, where mountains, chairs,
        windows, meadows,
Lighthouses, graffiti, trees, sand dunes, power stations
        intermingle, offering
The viewer many potential routes through a sometimes
        considerable length
Of scenery. Take for instance the boats, the jetty, the sweeping
        path to the volcano,
The chapel on the hill. Sometimes some words of the print of
        the newspaper support

Are left visible, though more often than not they are veiled or
    totally obscured.

Typically, his day starts with a read of the newspaper.
    The Guardian, specifically.
He scans for things he might use between reading and
    looking until
Something, whether photograph or text, engages him –
    an area of brickwork, say, or of
Repeated prepositions. So he pulls out the page, thinks, and
    paints something on
The something on the page; thinks again, paints again. He
    likes the way newspaper
Gets wrinkled and puckered when painted on, and gives
    what's been obliterated
Incidental texture. Thing after thing he follows what he thinks
    they want to become.

Seeing I take *The Guardian*, I think I'll try that too. See where
    it takes me.
So this morning – the 11th of May 2019 – I open the paper at
    random at a feature
On the Venice Biennale, where I read about Julie Mehretu,
    'whose paintings
Often use newspaper images as their source, but overpainted …
    so that
Their original material becomes obscured'. I take this as a
    favourable omen to write

Toward Venice, in the form of Canaletto's *The Stonemason's Yard*,
    a picture
I'd been always taken by. From now on I can take it as a
    palimpsest to write upon.

And what a different take on Venice is *The Stonemason's Yard*
    from the standard
Canaletto Grand Tourist view: those magnificent regattas on
    the Grand Canal –
Golden pageantry, the gorgeous barges and the glittering
    palazzi – no, this is
Almost Dutch, attentive to the everyday, the seemingly
    authoritative title a misnomer:
The view is of the Campo San Vidal, the 'yard' a temporary
    set-up for the repair of
The nearby church (not seen in the picture) of San Vidal,
    though on Google Maps it lies immediately
Behind the viewer. The church across the canal – it is indeed
    the Grand Canal! –

Is that of Santa Maria della Carità, whose campanile collapsed
    on 17th March 1744
And was never rebuilt. I'm thinking what a clatter the bells
    must have made
As they fell, when suddenly, the *ting-ting* of your incoming
    Fonacab 'taxi dispatched' text!
I close the laptop. Twenty minutes later we're in the waiting
    room. It takes an hour

THE BREATH OF CONSOLATION

Before we're seen, but now I'm seated in the La-Z-Boy recliner,
    hooked up
To the drip: a 1115ml infusion over 60 minutes. I've brought
    along a little Thames
And Hudson Canaletto pocket book by Antonio Paolucci to
    pass the time.

I look at it from time to time. There's an LED display with a
    digital countdown on
The trolley but I have to look over my shoulder for it. In any
    event it issues
An almost inaudible murmur I imagine measuring the chemo
    trickling down…
Dozing a little, I hear it entering my ear canal… *cannula,*
    cannula, Canaletto, Canaletto…
I open my eyes and there you are, looking at me. I say, Can you
    get the Muji pen
And notebook from my jacket pocket? And write this down?
    You do. *My writing hand*
Is out of action due to the cannula in the wrist through which the
    chemo flows.

The LED begins to flash and beep. Chemo's nearly over, just
    00.05 on the clock, then
We're out. But first I have to pee! The chemo fairly makes you
    go. Now much relieved
And in the taxi home, I'm looking at the picture in the pocket
    book. Barely three

Inches by four, but what a world of characters and things
    implying time – the gondoliers
Who ply their measured pole from quay to quay; the time it
    takes for the distaff woman
On the balcony to spin a length of yarn; or for the stooping
    woman to draw
Water from the well. As for the workmen chipping away amid
    the rubble at the marble

Bit by bit – see how the white stone is reflected by the high,
    dazzling bell tower
In the background to the right – are they paid by piece or by
    time? From the shadows
Cast it looks like mid-morning. How long is it since the cock
    first crew – there,
Perched resplendent on that window sill, looking east from
    the left of the frame?
The two lines of washing on the far bank, will they be dry by
    noon? The pot plants
On an upper balcony, in what sequence planted? Over
    everything and everyone
The bell-strokes of the campanile of Santa Maria della Carità
    proclaim the proper time.

Then there is the deep time of the City of Venice, floating on
    sleech on a city of stilts.
The stone, how long did it take to quarry and ship from
    Istria to here,

To say nothing of its archaeology? Paint layers at another end
    of the temporal spectrum:
Now I'm looking on the internet at this magnified 400x
    cross-section sample
Of a microscopic flake of terracotta building: lead white, red
    and orange ochres,
Naples yellow, red lake, and some black. A scintilla of Venetian
    sky: lead white,
Vermilion, Prussian blue and yellow earth. The Prussian blue
    has faded over time –

Everything infused by time and marble dust! But look at
    the toddler in the foreground who,
Fallen backwards on his bottom, has just released this elegant,
    sparkling arc of pee!
His mother commiserates; he'd been doing so well at the
    staggering toward her
Open arms. He'll learn in time how many steps to take before
    whatever end
He had in mind; and I, however long it takes to write this
    poem, whatever it might be.
For here we are again in Hopefield, looking through the green
    chain-link fencing
At the big yellow JCB. And as for what they're going to build
    there, we can't wait to see.

John Constable,
Study of Clouds, 1822

'The sound of water escaping from mill dams, etc., willows, old rotten planks,
Slimy posts and brickwork, I love such things,' said Constable. Also, trees and wind
And clouds reflected in the water, as shown by his limpid
    Water-meadows at Salisbury.
His father owned watermills and windmills; he understood weather from childhood.
Of hail squalls in spring he had this to say: 'The clouds accumulate in very large masses,
And from their loftiness seem to move but slowly; immediately on these large clouds
Appear numerous opaque patches, which are only small clouds passing rapidly
Before them. Those floating much nearer the earth may perhaps fall in with
A stronger current of wind, which drives them with greater rapidity from light to shade
Through the lanes of the clouds; hence they are called by wind-millers and sailors, *Messengers*,
And always portend bad weather.' Therefore Constable learned the craft of chiaroscuro.
Ten years ago it was your going through what had to be gone through. First the little blip,
Then the bigger blip. We'd scan the clouds for whatever augury they bore, clouds
That bloom and dim from marble sheen to darks of silver at the edges, in the throes of being

And becoming. Shown what showed on the screen, we
              wondered, what do we know of
Our bodies, the internal country undiscovered until now,
              and then not understood? Now
It has befallen me to go through what will be, we gaze into
              the clouds and listen to the sound
Of water in the Waterworks … I open a book to see what
              Constable recorded one day on
Hampstead Heath: '31st Sepr 10 – 11 o'clock morning looking
              Eastward a gentle wind to the East' –
The moving cumulus caught on the fly between hand and eye?
              Study, as in 'an act of learning'?
Let's say a happenstance of Constable and cloud, the final
              picture uninterpretable –
Quasi-shapely, cauliflower-plump, with just a hint of dark
              top right to prove the chiaroscuro.

First Light:
A selection of poems (2015)

Philip Hodgins
(Australian writer 1959–1995)

In the immediate aftermath of my cancer diagnosis a fragment of a poem hovered at the edge of my consciousness, refusing to budge. "The cause of death is in the blood and bone. It breeds in the past, feeds on the future." These lines spoke so clearly about blood cancer that I longed to unlock the memory. However hard I tried, though, no poet's name nor even a trace of a context came back to me. Months passed and I all but gave up. Then, in reading's lovely, serendipitous way, I chanced upon the poet and my original source again. Leafing through Clive James's collection of essays *The Meaning of Recognition*, I rediscovered a glorious tribute to the Australian writer Philip Hodgins. James's eulogy, with its tantalising mention of Hodgins's Irish roots, had first aroused my curiosity back in the mid-2000s. I recall being struck by extracts from Hodgins's work and wanting to read more. Shocked to discover that no Irish public library north or south held any, I tried but failed to source a title for Cavan Library. Close to twenty years later and still no Irish public library holds even one collection by Philip Hodgins. Luckily, the Australian Poetry Library website gave me access to his poetry as I waited for the collection *First Light* to arrive from New York. Reading Hodgins's poems through the lens of a chronic leukaemia diagnosis was an intensely moving experience. He powerfully articulates the grim realities of living with and slowly dying from a chronic and incurable blood cancer.

Although Philip Hodgins saw himself as an entirely Australian poet, there is evidence of a keen awareness of his Irish roots in his poetic output. His parents were born and grew up in Northern Ireland and emigrated in 1951 to Australia, eventually establishing a small dairy farm near the small town of Katandra West in Victoria. Born in 1959, Hodgins was an only child whose childhood and adolescent experiences of farming life shaped him. A defining moment came with the distressing loss of the family farm when he was nineteen. In 1983, aged just twenty-four, he was diagnosed with chronic myeloid leukaemia. Given three years to live, he survived for nearly twelve, eventually dying in 1995 aged thirty-six. Although he had been writing poetry from a young age, the shock of his diagnosis was the catalyst that drove him to become a fully-fledged poet.

The Australian poet and critic Les Murray was spot on when he stated that Hodgins writes "truly straight and plain". There is nothing pretentious in how Hodgins uses poetic language. His laconic and understated style marries with a clarity and a directness that make his poetry genuinely accessible. Nevertheless, there is no mistaking his mastery of language and form, nor the meticulous attention with which he forged his work. There is so much for the reader to enjoy, from the carefully considered choice of words and rhyming schemes to the wit, humour and irony that is in evidence throughout his body of work. That sense of irony is ubiquitous, present not only in the poetry itself but also in poem and collection titles. He has an eye for a telling detail and an uncanny knack for writing unforgettable endings. He is, it should be said, no romantic: poem after poem paints an experience of loss and grief that is shocking, even frightening at times.

For a time following his diagnosis, leukaemia and mortality were all that he could write about. His first two poetry collections, *Blood and Bone* and *Down the Lake With Half a Chook*, were, as the poet himself stated, a way of confronting the tragedy that had befallen him. The anguish that pours out of what are often referred to as his "death" poems is palpable. A fierce truthfulness in these accomplished and sophisticated early poems resonates deeply with the reader. We experience his terror, vulnerability, self-pity and isolation. We are with him as he senses the unease of friends who can offer only platitudes. We empathise as he agonises over the suffering that his terminal illness is inflicting on his parents. Hodgins's harrowing 'needle' poems capture that claustrophobic sense of being removed from ordinary life and entrapped in an alien environment dominated by the presence and sounds of machines. In his hospital world needles are ever-present and he imbues them with a sense of menace. Hodgins's striking and original imagery is drawn from his formative years on the family dairy farm. The land and his childhood memories provided a deep well of images that he transformed into powerful metaphors for cancer and mortality. Animal deaths feature time and again. In the poem 'Shooting the Dogs', a memory of having to kill the family dogs for practical reasons becomes a meditation on death and how random and brutal it often is. Hodgins drives home his message in his last lines.

> Each time the gravel slid off the shovel
> it sounded like something
> trying to hang on by its nails.

It is a chilling reminder that we have no control over our own death. The natural drive in all living things to hold onto life at any cost is acknowledged. We may be prepared to do anything to survive but when the moment of death arrives, all our struggles to resist the grave are destined to come to nought. Every human being must find a way to accept this truth. Hodgins was a master at layering meaning in his poems. 'Shooting the Dogs' is also a meditation on the heart-breaking struggles of poor farmers trying to eke out a living and survive in desperate, often hopeless, economic circumstances.

There is a terrible beauty in Hodgins's cancer poetry. Evan Jones, an Australian poet and academic, drew a striking comparison between Hodgins's work and that of the great First World War poets. It is easy to see why. Hodgins knew what it was to be mortally wounded, utterly vulnerable and faced with the nearness of death in what should have been the prime of his life. His articulation of human suffering in such extreme circumstances is evocative, intense and wholly authentic. In finding a way to voice his own experience with terminal cancer so brilliantly, he communicates meaningfully with readers and provides a means for others to make sense of their own cancer struggles.

After eighteen months, Hodgins had, in his own words, 'written out' the disease. He consciously moved on to become a prolific writer on other themes. Critically acclaimed for his pastoral poetry, he also wrote passionately about Australian Rules Football and family life. A regular contributor to Australian newspapers, anthologies and literary journals, his work appeared in *The New Yorker* and *the Paris Review*. One of my favourite Hodgins poems has nothing whatsoever to do with cancer or mortality. 'Milk Cream Butter' is a sensuous portrayal of a daily dairy farm ritual. It is a delightful poem, reminiscent of the early work of Seamus Heaney, another Ulster farmer's son. That Hodgins found it possible to move beyond his "cancer" poems and focus so successfully on other themes is, as Clive James rightly points out, an incredible achievement. He made every effort to transcend a disease that never loosened its grip on his short life. He wrote about rural realities and the way in which the landscape is shaped by, and in turn shapes, human activity. He had no illusions about the tough and unforgiving nature of farming life and was critical of questionable farming practices that played a part in damaging the environment and resulted in the mistreatment of animals. Knowing that exposure to herbicides and pesticides was a possible explanation for his cancer coloured his unsentimental view of farming. It is impossible not to shudder when you read the poems 'At the Sheep-Parasite Field Day' and 'Second Thoughts on The Georgics'.

> I was drenched to the bone with DDT,
> They told me to have a good long shower
> but I still felt sick as a dog later on.

Overhanging all of his poetic output is the ever-darkening shadow of his cancer diagnosis, recurring hospital treatments and devastating prognosis. Despite his determination to move away from serious illness as a major theme, a sense of foreboding permeates much of his writing. In fact, some of his finest metaphorical poems about cancer and death are found in the pastoral collections. In *Up on All Fours* the poem 'The Pier' addresses the insidious way in which leukaemia undermines and eventually destroys the human body. It has a quiet calmness about the inevitability of approaching death that lingers in the reader's mind.

Hodgins's last collection, *Things Happen*, was published posthumously. In his final work he not only continues to integrate his principal themes of serious illness and rural life but also speaks directly about cancer and mortality once again. Hodgins's delight in words and meanings is one of the pleasures to be found in his work. I love the way one of his earliest poems, 'Room 1 Ward 10 West 23/11/83', is echoed and amplified twelve years later in one of his very last, 'Wordy Wordy Numb Numb'. Both are moving meditations on the importance of language and meaning, and on our inescapable mortality. Among many unforgettable poems in *Things Happen*, 'A House in the Country' stands out. In it, a home riddled with termites becomes a symbol for a body invaded by cancer cells. Like the termites, the cancer cells burrow in, undetectable until it is too late, and slowly rot the blood and the bone from within. There is no cure, no effective way of dislodging the invader. The sickening image of "the bloated queen" busy producing more and more termites is powerful. The sense of fear and the realisation that there is no escape engulfs reader as well as writer in these, his final poems.

Hodgins twists the pervasive symbolism of light as a bearer of goodness, purity, life, warmth and hope into something altogether different. In 'More Light, More Light' it becomes a negative symbol, sickly, lifeless, ruthlessly exposing the awful reality of serious illness and fast-approaching death. The shift is jarring yet effective. So too are the subtle references to Goethe's last words and to Anthony Hecht's famous poem of almost the same title, 'More Light! More Light!', which is regarded as one of the finest poems about the Holocaust. Like Hecht, Hodgins seems to be telling us that it is not only the poet's right but also his duty to create poetic art from horrifying and traumatic realities.

A true original, Hodgins was able to fuse key themes – farming life, serious illness, loss, and mortality – into extraordinary and deeply moving poetry that is, ironically, teeming with life. It is a testament to his brilliance that he enables us to enter fully into his experiences. There is a depth to Hodgins's work that reveals itself slowly and is all the more satisfying for that. My hope is that his inclusion in this book will win him new readers who will find solace in his words. It would be thrilling if it also prompts Irish public libraries to stock his poetry and academics to research how Hodgins's Ulster roots impacted on his writing.

Room 1 Ward 10 West 23/11/83
(first published in Blood and Bone, *1986)*

Wordless afternoon
before my friends
for all their reasons
look in on me

They have time
to choose the words
they would
like me to hear

I am attached
to a dark
bag of blood
leaking near me

I have time
to choose the words
I am
likely to need

At twenty-four
there are many words
and this one
death

PHILIP HODGINS

A House in the Country
(first published in Things Happen, *1995)*

The first thing we knew about this hidden force
was when a crack appeared in the masonite
outside the children's bedroom, starting from
up under one end of the windowsill
and taking a jagged diagonal course
that led down to the bottom of the wall
as if it were a chart of our bad luck.

With burglar care I used a jemmy to pry
the two large pieces of this puzzle off
their web-filled grid of noggins and studs
and saw immediately the tell-tale dry
mud tubes that were plastered to several of
the concrete stumps, those conduits termites make
to get out of the earth and into the goods.

The first stud I prodded buckled and split
and something hard to focus on, a sprinkling
of tiny cloned albino movement, split
and dispersed, and was followed by even more
when I levered the stud apart, the panic of
a light-shy mass, so translucently pale
they looked as if they weren't fully formed.

Again I rowed the jemmy through a stud
and got the same result, more spillage
from what was now no longer a closed circuit,
and with a teenage vandal's feeling of

THE BREATH OF CONSOLATION

futility and despair I smashed the mud
conduits on the stumps within my reach,
releasing a more concentrated flow.

I gazed at this miniature apocalypse
of countless termites writhing in exposure,
no doubt programmed to crave the opposite
of Goethe, who had cried *More light! More light!*
and as the seconds dropped away as small
and uniform as termites a feeling burrowed
into me as bad as if I had cancer.

I thought about the treatment this would mean:
those poisons, vile as chemotherapy,
that they'd have to spray all round the place,
a pile of new timber, tin caps between
the bearers and the stumps, and hours, maybe days
spent wandering the paddocks like prospectors
on the off-chance that we'd find the nest.

Somewhere out there, sealed in a slightly warm
and humid city was the bloated queen,
unable to move, surrounded by her swarm
of attendants, an evil sausage producing more
and more termites that would eat our home.
I set off at a fast walk, worried about
what was going on underneath my feet.

PHILIP HODGINS

Blood Connections
(first published in Things Happen, *1995)*

"Is that an Ulster accent I detect?"
I'm lying on the trolley like a specimen
beside the leucophoresis machine.
The nurse regards me for a moment then
answers cautiously, "Yes, that's correct."
I tell her I'm Australian though my genes,
or most of them, originate from there
and she tells me how long she's been out here.
The red lights on the panel flash as if
it's not long till a bomb somewhere goes off.
She takes a lumen and my catheter
then pushes slowly so the lines connect
and saline comes to me from the machine.
We trade the names of Northern Irish towns
and find our mothers' home towns are the same:
so while she works on me I chat with her
around the edges of a heritage.
I tell her how my parents came out here
by ship in fifty-one and that my father
still gets his home-town paper by airmail
and knows the goings-on in Joycean detail.
The nurse unpacks a needle and a line.
"We're probably related," she almost jokes,
but wary of which side I'm on she looks
me in the eye, just momentarily,
a look that asks, "Are your folks killing mine?"
The tourniquet is tightened to a grip
and veins rise up in long soft flexed protest.

THE BREATH OF CONSOLATION

I watch the needle hovering over me.
It's big. It goes in slowly and it hurts.
I watch the blood run through the line. It's fast.
The machine begins to pump. The pain gets worse.
I think of saying something but the vein bursts.
Inside my elbow it begins to spasm blue.
The machine shuts down and switches on a light.
The needle is withdrawn, the site bound tight.
The muscles in my arm begin to spasm too.
And then the blind convulsions spread
all through my body, carried there by blood.
The nurse tells me the name of this reaction
and fills a big syringe with valium,
undoes my catheter, makes a new connection
and pushes in the calming drug. "No harm,"
she says, in the accent of my childhood home,
and goes around to try the other arm.

PHILIP HODGINS

Wordy Wordy Numb Numb
(first published in Things Happen, *1995)*

Death.
Now there's a word.
He wrote it down.

It didn't take up much space.
You could say it was discreet,
and patient.

He couldn't remember
the first time he'd heard it.
It seemed to have been always there,

like something he owned
as a kind of right or inheritance.
But he wasn't sure if this was true.

He liked the way it rhymed
with breath,
its natural opposite.

He liked it for many reasons,
and because of that
he wrote it down many times

in many different contexts
finding that it had
all sorts of meanings.

THE BREATH OF CONSOLATION

Later on, when words had passed,
he backed it up
by dying.

One thing
he had always remembered
was the arrogance of health,

those dumb days
when nothing can touch you,
when death is just one

of the familiar short words:
sun, moon, tree, bread, wine, house, love ...
you know them,

each one worn smooth
as a river stone
with the flow of language

and death the odd one out,
not so much worn smooth
as numb.

Better not to think about it then
and come back to it later
when it comes back to you

like an unpaid debt
gathering interest
infinitely greater than what was lent.

All of Us:
The Collected Poems (1996)

Raymond Carver

(*American writer 1938–1988*)

For many Irish readers the short story form is a natural home, familiar and loved. Little wonder then that Raymond Carver was on my radar solely for his masterly short story collections. Until, that is, I stumbled upon his poetry for the first time in the compulsively readable Lifelines series of poetry anthologies. That initial encounter in the 1990s with just a handful of his poems – 'Happiness', 'Gravy', 'Late Fragment' and 'What the Doctor Said' – made a powerful impression. Here was a poet within reach of general readers attracted to, if also a little intimidated by, the world of poetry. However, it took a cancer diagnosis and the idea for this book to finally prod me into seeking out his body of poetic work.

Read for the first time at the very start of the research process, *All of Us* left an indelible mark. As months stretched into years, the work of many poets passed through my hands and difficult choices had to be made but Raymond Carver's inclusion was never in question. The only difficulty was deciding which of his poetry books to select. It was tempting to opt for Carver's final book of poems, *A New Path to the Waterfall*, written as he approached death and containing many of the most appropriate poems for this collection. However, the cumulative effect of reading all of his poetic work is so much more than the sum of its parts. Forged in dire life experiences and haunted by death, his poetry is suffused with guilt, loss and sorrow. Yet it is his acute awareness of the preciousness of life, of the happiness to be found in everyday living, and of the personal responsibility to make the most of every minute, that reverberates and lodges in the reader's heart. Carver's juxtaposition of darkness, desolation and misery with happiness, gratitude and joy endows his poetry with startling power. It is as if he has somehow uncovered the secret of life and shared that knowledge in a poetic language that rings with clarity and truth. *All of Us* displays Carver's skill as a master storyteller, muddying the line between prose and poetry, making it unique and accessible but also exhilarating.

Carver's personal story is intimately connected with his poetry. In his last interviews he stated that he viewed his life experiences as an emotional reservoir for his writing. Just fifty when he died, Carver considered that he had lived two distinct lives. The first was full of darkness, desolation and despair. Carver was born into poverty, raised in a dysfunctional family and married with two children at twenty. Mired in a succession of soul-destroying blue-collar jobs as he dealt with debt and bankruptcies, his obsession with writing remained constant. In *All of Us* he writes movingly of a transformative moment in his teenage years when, thanks to the casual generosity of a stranger, he was gifted a copy of *Poetry* magazine and, with it, the knowledge that a career in writing was a legitimate possibility. Throughout the 1960s Carver strove for an academic education and participated in creative writing workshops at various universities whilst struggling to support his family. The signs of a writer of substance emerging were clear, although Carver was only able to write fitfully. By the late 1960s, his work was gaining critical regard. For instance, his story 'Will You Please Be Quiet, Please?' was included in *The Best American Short Stories 1967*. By this time, however, alcoholism had taken hold and it became the biggest obstacle to his writing life. As the 1970s progressed he did little writing, was regularly hospitalised for alcoholism and his marriage was failing. Alcoholism eventually nearly killed him.

Carver's life was transformed in the late 1970s when he stopped drinking for good, separated from his first wife and then met and fell in love with the poet Tess Gallagher. Sober, with academic work and grants finally providing a measure of financial security and stability, and with time at last to focus on his writing, Carver could begin his 'second life'. Over the next ten years, he flourished both professionally and personally. Success and critical recognition on a scale unimaginable during his dark years followed, together with lasting personal happiness. Lauded for his short stories, it is sometimes forgotten that he began his literary career as a poet and wrote both poetry and prose in tandem throughout his life. Carver refused to be pigeon-holed as a writer of just one form and produced most of his poetic work over the course of his last ten years, resulting in the publication of three poetry collections. A lifetime heavy smoker, he once described himself as "a cigarette with a body attached to it". Yet, a lung cancer diagnosis in September 1987, which was followed by the removal of two thirds of one lung, was still a deeply shocking moment for Carver. The reprieve that followed treatment proved short-lived. A brain tumour diagnosis in March 1988 led to seven weeks of intense brain radiation. By June 1988, cancer had again been found in his lungs. Faced with such a devastating prognosis, Carver chose to keep writing, determined to utilise every minute of remaining life. With the support of Tess Gallagher, Carver's wonderful last poetry collection, *A New Path to the Waterfall,* was completed and published posthumously. Carver described his poetry as "a small good thing". For the reader, it is an intensely moving literary accomplishment. *All of Us* is an extraordinary and consoling gift, most especially for those living and dying with cancer.

It is difficult, if not impossible, to generalise about Carver's poetry. Long narrative and confessional poems sit side by side with lyrical work and even a little prose. The delicate blend of his own poetry with extracts from writers spiritually important to him including Anton Chekhov, Czeslaw Milosz and Jaroslave Seifert works brilliantly. Events and memories are recalled together with the moods and emotions they invoked. Moving through the collection is an unsettling experience for the reader. Carver manages to surprise but also unnerve us. Not just from poem to poem but often within poems the subtle twists in mood, tone and subject matter are unexpected, as with 'The Schooldesk' (written in Ireland) and 'Earwigs'.

He lifts the reader's heart with poems celebrating life, love, friendship and the beauty of the natural world. In 'Near Klamath' and 'Wind' for example, Carver captures the sheer delight of simply being alive to the wonders of nature and the joy of fishing in the company of friends. In 'After Reading Two Towns in Provence' he reminds us of the pleasure and consolation of losing oneself in literature. 'Happiness' and 'My Work' are two beautifully observed poems suffused with appreciation and a heightened sense of gratitude for the way life brings unexpected moments of happiness. Tenderness and love ooze out of the many poems written about his relationship with Tess. Carver clearly appreciated the enormous gift of having such a truthful, loving and fulfilled relationship to rely on, most especially as death approached. He both honours and celebrates that love in poem after poem.

Nonetheless, the spectre of his first life is ever present in harrowing images of alcoholism, domestic violence and dysfunctional families. The lifetime burden of damaged family relationships is captured in many poems including 'Miracle', 'To My Daughter', 'My Daughter and Apple Pie' and 'On an Old Photograph of My Son'. Using memories and anecdotes, Carver slowly builds a sense of not only the agony but also the ecstasy experienced over a lifetime. As he weaves together dark poetry with light-filled and tender work, he encapsulates the conflicted nature of human life as it is rather than as we would wish it to be. He also nudges us to remember that there is always hope and it is possible to rise above suffering and survive.

The menacing presence of death can be felt right from the start of the collection. In early poems such as 'Woolworth's 1954' and 'Fear' the poet struggles to even write the word, yet a sense of death pervades his poetry. It is when we reach the final poems, written as he struggled to come to terms with his impending demise, that Carver's stoicism and inner strength are plainly in sight. The cluster of last poems – 'What the Doctor Said', 'Gravy', 'No Need', 'Through the Boughs', and 'Late Fragment' – have a purity and intensity that is moving and extraordinarily powerful. Carver strikes a delicate balance between loving life and accepting death. There is a sense of peace, even of quiet celebration as he writes his farewells, giving thanks for his life whilst mourning it at the same time. It is as if he is gently showing us how best to die. There was never any doubt in my mind that the poetry section had to end with Carver's 'Late Fragment'. What a consoling legacy he has bequeathed to those of us who love literature, and how blessed are those readers who encounter his poetry for the first time here. Take heart from what Carver has to say to us.

What the Doctor Said

He said it doesn't look good
he said it looks bad in fact real bad
he said I counted thirty-two of them on one lung before
I quit counting them
I said I'm glad I wouldn't want to know
about any more being there than that
he said are you a religious man do you kneel down
in forest groves and let yourself ask for help
when you come to a waterfall
mist blowing against your face and arms
do you stop and ask for understanding at those moments
I said not yet but I intend to start today
he said I'm really sorry he said
I wish I had some other kind of news to give you
I said Amen and he said something else
I didn't catch and not knowing what else to do
and not wanting him to have to repeat it
and me to have to fully digest it
I just looked at him
for a minute and he looked back it was then
I jumped up and shook hands with this man who'd just given me
something no one else on earth had ever given me
I may even have thanked him habit being so strong

Gravy

No other word will do. For that's what it was. Gravy.
Gravy, these past ten years.
Alive, sober, working, loving and
being loved by a good woman. Eleven years
ago he was told he had six months to live
at the rate he was going. And he was going
nowhere but down. So he changed his ways
somehow. He quit drinking! And the rest?
After that it was *all* gravy, every minute
of it, up to and including when he was told about,
well, some things that were breaking down and
building up inside his head. "Don't weep for me,"
he said to his friends. "I'm a lucky man.
I've had ten years longer than I or anyone
expected. Pure gravy. And don't forget it."

Through the Boughs

Down below the window, on the deck, some ragged-looking
birds gather at the feeder. The same birds, I think,
that come every day to eat and quarrel. *Time was, time was,*
they cry and strike at each other. It's nearly time, yes.
The sky stays dark all day, the wind is from the west and
won't stop blowing ... Give me your hand for a time. Hold on
to mine. That's right, yes. Squeeze hard. Time was we
thought we had time on our side. *Time was, time was,*
those ragged birds cry.

Late Fragment

And did you get what
you wanted from this life, even so?
I did.
And what did you want?
To call myself beloved, to feel myself
beloved on the earth.

PART 4

Short Stories and Novellas

Introduction

The short story holds a special place in my heart, as it does for most Irish readers. It is imprinted in our DNA, after all, passed down from generation to generation, forever a strong presence in our lives. The roots of our deep love lie in a rich storytelling tradition, a childhood diet of Irish sagas and folktales, and the classroom presence of short stories by Irish masters of the genre. The richness and diversity of Irish short stories laid a solid foundation for encounters with classics by Russian, French and English writers. The world of the North American short story, particularly those written by women, opened up later in my reading life and cast a spell that has never been broken. Something magical happens when a writer distils a story into a highly concentrated and intense form, whether it is a short story or a novella. The genre's very essence, its unique characteristics, makes it ideally suited for those living and dying with cancer.

So, what are those characteristics? The most obvious is also the most deceptive. A short story is easily approached and can be read in one sitting. It grabs the reader's attention immediately. The real pleasure however lies in how it slows reading down and demands close and undivided attention. It is remarkably easy to lose yourself completely in a short story. It is the prose form that is closest to poetry and is dense with compressed meaning. Figuring out that meaning requires the reader to pause, question and consider. The reader is compelled to quieten down the reading process in order to take things in. Above all, the reader has to listen attentively to what the writer has chosen to reveal and what has been withheld, and why. Ambiguous endings are a staple of the short story form, freeing readers to infer conclusions for themselves. It is as if the writer is saying to the reader – over to you, now. Make of it what you will. Perfectly crafted short stories are spellbinding and always true to the complexities of human life.

In addition, the themes that dominate in short stories are the very themes that are of primary concern for the seriously ill: isolation; loneliness; failures of human connection; the inner struggle for self-understanding; and the desire to bring coherence to a complex mishmash of human emotions. The ambiguities and complexities that haunt an individual life are powerfully articulated in the short story form and so, universal experiences are illuminated in fresh and often surprising ways. The reader comes away thinking differently and seeing the world afresh.

Undoubtedly, the genre's most pleasing characteristics are its sheer beauty and its diversity. The short story is an inherently innovative and creative literary space that embraces complexities and resists easy solutions. So much is expressed within tight confines. Meticulously crafted and thematically rich stories abound, brimming with poetic language, acutely observed detail, exceptional characterisation and unforgettable imagery. There are good reasons why we gravitate towards poetic work in challenging times. Like poetry, great short stories connect and resonate with the battered and bruised soul. They give us an imaginative space to retreat to. Our minds are never as alive as when we are engrossed in the work of a great poet or short story writer. There is an intimacy to the reading experience that is in itself consoling. Short story writers and poets are uniquely capable of giving voice to the complex truths of the cancer experience, all the while reminding us of the commonality of experiences and our shared fragility.

One of the secret pleasures of working on this anthology has been breaking my own predetermined rules when the material demanded it. I tried to be professional and objective throughout, researching and reading as widely as possible. I never wavered in my desire to discover the finest short story writing that explored relevant themes from various standpoints and in a wide variety of writing styles. Fourteen stories, rather than the ten originally planned, made the cut. All are absolute gems and will speak meaningfully to the reader with cancer. When I took a step back to consider the final selection, I recognised that my personal taste is loudly proclaimed, perhaps more so here than in any other section. Seven women writers are included. Feminist values and the struggle for social justice are important elements in the works chosen. North American short stories predominate.

Stories by critically lauded and award-winning writers (including Nobel, Booker, and Pulitzer prize-winners) sit cheek-by-jowl with works of excellence from debut collections. Five short stories are from one collection by a masterful short story writer. To my shame, Lucia Berlin was unknown to me when I started this project but is now beloved. Two classic and revered novellas feature.

INTRODUCTION

Published in 1886 and 1960, respectively, both are as fresh and original as any of the later work. Some stories have been widely anthologised whilst others are virtually unheard of, even amongst avid short story readers. Cancer and mortality are central preoccupations and yet it is life that is celebrated in works that radiate compassion and humanity.

It was exciting to find so many parallels, intersections, and connections between the chosen stories. Across different cultures, time periods, and writing styles, it is as if the writers have listened to and absorbed the imaginative approaches of earlier masters. A case in point is Thom Jones's 'I Want to Live!'. No one could miss its similarities to Tolstoy's *The Death of Ivan Ilyich*. I was constantly reminded of Alice Munro's 'Floating Bridge' as I read Mary Costello's 'Little Disturbances'. Another striking and recurring element is the fusion of the fictional and the autobiographical. Lucia Berlin, Lorrie Moore and Thom Jones have transformed stories anchored in personal experiences into works of emotional intensity and startling power. Finally, the gritty realism of those stories that confront the grim physical realities of cancer will no doubt resonate with the lived experiences of many readers.

The themes that dominate throughout are familiar territory for the seriously ill: the heightened need for empathy and connection; the true nature of close relationships and of family life; the struggle with inner turmoil; the desire for self-understanding; the urge to make sense of a previously unexamined life; the fear of approaching death; and the fierce desire to live. This multiplicity of themes is dealt with so creatively that the genre feels tailor-made for any great cancer literature lifeline.

Although all fourteen stories stand alone and are perfectly complete, it was satisfying to include works that are part of a cycle of interlinked stories. The attraction of such short story sequences is clear to readers who love books like Joyce's *Dubliners*. So, venture beyond the individual stories from *Union Street* and *Olive, Again* and dive into the complete works to enrich your reading experience.

A lifelong love affair with the short story has convinced me that it is the prose form that comes closest to literary perfection. The selected works exemplify the absolute best that the genre has to offer. Every story shines a light on specific aspects of the cancer experience, providing haunting portrayals of the complexities and challenges of living with cancer and at the edge of life and death. All fourteen stories are deeply affecting, delivering beauty, style and insight. My fervent hope is that readers will share my enthusiasm and find solace in this gathering of treasures by masters of the short story genre writing about cancer and mortality.

'Grief', 'Fool to Cry', 'Panteón de Dolores', 'Mama' and 'Wait a Minute'
from *A Manual for Cleaning Women* (2015)
Stories first published from the 1970s to the 1990s

Lucia Berlin
(American writer 1936–2004)

The discovery of Lucia Berlin's work was a moment of pure joy on my quest to find the finest short stories about the cancer experience. Berlin's career-spanning collection *A Manual for Cleaning Women* contains not one but five relevant short stories, any one of which could rightly claim a place in this anthology. All five explore the evolving relationship between two sisters brought together by a cancer diagnosis after years apart. Each story stands alone and perfectly complete, at a particular moment in time and with a specific focus. Berlin subtly alters the prism through which the sisters' lives are viewed with every story. Time periods shift significantly, as do geographic locations. As the narration moves fluidly and organically between present and past, the terrible legacy of a damaged childhood is laid bare and the sisters' radically different lifepaths come into view. Their enduring bond deepens and strengthens under the ever-increasing burden of terminal cancer. Taken together, these five interlocking stories can be read as a single, extended narrative of undeniable power and intensity. Berlin was a gifted and innovative writer, with a unique voice. Here, she delivers a riveting portrayal of two utterly believable women coming to terms with trauma, loss and death.

Her stories are full of colour and teaming with life even when the subject matter is bleak and desperately sad. Lydia Davis's foreword provides a wonderfully succinct yet comprehensive analysis of Berlin's writing, outlining the many reasons why she is so widely admired by critics and readers alike. Every story is anchored in Berlin's life experiences and personal memories which she transforms into glorious narrative. At first it appears to be haphazard storytelling, full of surprising twists and turns. It feels at times like the reader is swimming in a stream of consciousness where the narrator's memories, thoughts and feelings are flowing randomly. The reader often loses sight of where the story began and has little idea of where it might be heading. Nonetheless, it is always a compelling journey, described by a writer who radiates intelligence and compassion. Every story is dense with acutely observed details that bring both character and setting vibrantly to life. Her characterisation is unfailingly brilliant and her sympathetic and non-judgmental approach makes the behaviour of even the most dislikeable characters understandable. Berlin's peripatetic life ensured that place was really important to her and her settings are palpably real – every location buzzes with colour, sights, sounds and cultural differences.

Her style is direct but also seductive, reaching out and hooking the reader, mind and heart. Not one word is wasted. A subtle sense of humour enlivens the darkest moments. There are numerous laugh-out-loud instances created by her outrageously good comedic timing. As each story reaches its end, however, the writer's serious intent becomes clear. Every single incident and memory recounted have had purpose. The seeming naturalness of her writing masks just how skilfully and meticulously crafted her work is. Meaning is often revealed in exceptional final lines. As a writer of both style and substance, Berlin takes her personal story of caring for her dying sister and transforms it. The result is a razor-sharp study of the devastating impact of terminal cancer, and of the existential questions we all wrestle with when faced with life-threatening illness. Berlin's writing rings with truth.

We meet the sisters for the first time in the story **'Grief'**. The setting is a Mexican coastal resort and our initial impression of the sisters is formed by a retired German holidaymaker. Mrs. Wacher (a characteristically witty name choice) is naturally curious about two women who are lost in each other's company and talk incessantly. The younger sister's tearful episodes fuel her curiosity. Berlin paints an instantly recognisable resort scene with the usual mix of behaviours of humans at play. Her penchant for witty similes is immediately evident. Mrs. Wacher is soon in cahoots with Mrs Lewis, a like-minded Canadian. Together they set out to find out all they can about the women. It is through their antics that we learn the bare bones of the sisters' stories. The younger sister, Sally, is in her forties, married and living in Mexico City with her three children. She has had a mastectomy and is due to start radiation therapy. Dolores is in her fifties with four grown sons and works as a nurse in California. Their mother has recently died and the sisters haven't seen each other for twenty years. Berlin strikes a graceful balance in the story, alternating between the gossips' observations and the sisters' dialogue mingled with Dolores's thoughts and memories.

When the sisters move centre stage, we learn the real reason for Sally's tears. It is not cancer nor their mother's death, as the gossips suppose, but a husband's betrayal. Sally has been abandoned after twenty years for a younger, pregnant woman. In these early interchanges between the sisters the childhood pattern of their relationship is re-established. So too is the unerring ability of siblings to hit where it will hurt most. As they argue about the possibility of Sally's cancer returning, Sally resorts to a devastating putdown that recurs through all five stories:

> "You are so cold. Sometimes you are as cruel as Mama." Dolores said nothing. Her greatest fear, that she was like her mother. Cruel, a drunkard.

Whilst Sally's problems are openly discussed, Dolores hides a heavy secret. The shame of her alcoholism is amplified by the memories of their mother's dark history with the disease.

In a deeply touching sequence, Dolores uses every skill at her disposal, cajoling and bullying by turns, to force Sally into re-joining the land of the living. Sally is pushed into taking the crucial first steps towards acceptance of her scarred body. Dolores's efforts pay off and Sally dons a swimsuit, sunbathes, and eventually swims. As Sally begins to relax and enjoy the physical pleasures of sun and sea, her confidence builds and conversation flows. She speaks about the joy of her voluntary library work with impoverished children and Dolores reminds her that she has so much to live for. In stark contrast, Dolores has recently lost her nursing job because of her drinking, a fact she has not shared with her sister. Later, the subject of their damaged childhood comes up and Dolores suggests that it is time to talk about their mother. The first indications of their mother's reprehensible behaviour are given. Sally's deep pain resurfaces as she recalls being permanently cut out of her mother's life because she married a Mexican. Dolores attempts to repair her mother's image somewhat in Sally's eyes, hoping to ameliorate Sally's pain.

The last day of Sally's holiday arrives and Dolores continues to push Sally onwards through a healing process. Against her vehement objections, Sally goes scuba diving for the first time, with Dolores's former lover as her instructor. As the day unfolds and Sally learns the basics of scuba diving, Dolores is flooded with conflicting emotions. Humour, pathos, sisterly care, and self-disgust are all bound up in her thoughts and memories. Dolores's determination to help her sister heal from trauma is rewarded by Sally's ecstatic reaction. It is a response that reveals Sally's innate goodness and helps explain why she is so deeply loved by her older sister. Conversely, just as Sally is opening up and starting to embrace life again, Dolores is sinking under the weight of suppressed troubles which are festering away in her self-enforced silence. The dramatic changes in the sisters are revealed through Mrs. Wacher's observations. The dark shift in Dolores's frame of mind is matched by gathering storm clouds on the sister's last night together. In stark contrast, Sally is beginning to relish the joy of being alive.

Sally's face shone like a child's when the moonlight lit her.

It is an important image that, in modified form, recurs time and again and is in fact re-shaped for the final image in the last story. It is an indication of just how carefully crafted Berlin's work is. Sally's intense need to feel that her mother loved her despite all the evidence to the contrary sparks the last serious conversation of their holiday. Rather than telling Sally the truth – that her mother mocked Sally's sweetness and considered her a fool – Dolores lies, spinning a fairy tale of a loving mother watching over her young daughter, unseen. The reader begins to understand that Dolores's protective maternal instincts lie at the root of the tender bond between the sisters. After sweetly revealing the sisters' renewed bond, Berlin plunges us into the dark reality of Dolores's painful and carefully hidden alcoholic world. It is a master-class in great short storytelling.

When we next meet the sisters, in the story **'Fool to Cry'**, time has moved on. Sally's five-year remission has ended, cancer has returned, and maintenance chemotherapy is underway. It is clear to everyone that Sally is dying. Carlotta (in the first story called Dolores) has come to Mexico at her sister's request. Berlin plunges us straight into Sally's vibrant Mexican world of family, friends, and even a devoted lover. The warmth and naturalness of Mexican life is established and contrasted with American culture, firstly by the loving and tactile behaviour of Sally's two grown daughters and her fifteen-year-old son. After a night when a heavily medicated Sally sleeps through a series of tender family visits, the two sisters and Sally's son, Tino, go to a local café for morning coffee.

Frequented by Sally for years, the café is a place that leaps from the page, showcasing Berlin's magical touch with both settings and characters. The reader feels fully present, like an unseen observer sitting at an outer table watching all the comings and goings and eavesdropping on intimate conversations. We experience the loving interplay between Sally and her daughters, her powerful ex-husband, friends, café staff, and finally her lover. We hear a cherished old family story of a boy who fell in love with Carlotta on her twelfth birthday and has remained constant, sending flowers on her birthday every year for over forty years. With a subtle nod to the first story, we learn that the sisters have talked incessantly since Carlotta's arrival in Mexico. Sally has transformed in the intervening years and not in the way we might have expected for a dying woman.

> "Everyone knows she is dying, but she has never looked so beautiful or happy ... it is as if the sentence has been a gift ... She has come alive. She savors everything. She says whatever she wants, does what makes her feel good ... Little Sally, always meek and passive, in my shadow as a girl, in her husband's for most of her life. She is strong, radiant now, her zest is contagious."

The harsh reality of her condition is brought home, however, as Carlotta nurses her through the after-effects of the chemo. Sally's tears reflect her acute awareness of just how richly rewarding and happy her life now is, just as the end approaches. The sister's evolving relationship has matured and is clearly vitally important to their wellbeing. Berlin delivers a deeply touching account of how a sibling relationship, with the heft of shared genes, shared history, and mutual care and attention, can be so nurturing, sustaining and enriching.

THE BREATH OF CONSOLATION

In a sudden shift in the story's direction, Berlin arrives at Carlotta's fifty-fourth birthday and a planned lunch meeting with Basil, Carlotta's devoted admirer whom she has not seen since their youth. Before he arrives, Sally and Carlotta, together with Sally's daughters and Sally's two maids – de facto family members – watch a climactic episode of a tearjerker Mexican TV soap together. In a wonderfully feminine moment, replete with humour, the six women get caught up in the ridiculous plot and are moved to tears. Basil arrives and proves unequal to the sight of six women in tears and in various stages of undress, with Sally bald and wigless amongst them. This lunch date that has started so badly quickly descends into farce. Basil has become a loathsome and insensitive snob of a man. He is appalled by Sally's neighbourhood. When Carlotta explains the reason for Sally's baldness, he simply cannot comprehend how the women could be so giddy and so seemingly unaffected by Sally's cancer. Every attempt Carlotta makes to communicate is doomed. The quest for a suitable restaurant proves fruitless in a neighbourhood that Basil obviously abhors. Racist comments are followed by boastful talk of his children's achievements and of his wife's ability to keep servants in their place. He speaks with pride of his wealth, his summer home in Chile, his plans for retirement. Not content with boasting about his own life, he proceeds to dissect Carlotta's, pointing out how she has made a mess of it in a myriad of ways. She responds with spirit and humour to his invasive questions. When he pompously asks her what she has accomplished in life, this woman who has raised four sons, left everything to care for her sister, and lived life fully, can think of nothing at first. Her witty reply, when it comes, unexpectedly answers a question that has long been in the reader's mind.

> "'I haven't had a drink in three years,' I said.
> 'That's scarcely an accomplishment. That's like saying, 'I haven't murdered my mother.''
> 'Well, of course, there is that, too.' I smiled."

Carlotta then turns the tables on Basil with a question rooted in the nature of the boy Basil once was. His response is sad and revealing in ways that he could never understand. In Berlin's inimitable style, a stark reminder of what has become of Basil's poetic potential and, more generally, his human potential, is divulged during the drive back to Sally's home.

> "He recited all the deaths of people we had known, the financial and

marital failures of all my old boyfriends."

On reaching Sally's home, and for the first time since we were introduced to the sisters, it is Carlotta who cries. It is now Carlotta who urgently needs, seeks and receives comfort and support from Sally. The story ends with just one comment on the lunch meeting. It is all that is needed, as Sally and her daughters intuitively understand the devastating feelings of loss that have engulfed Carlotta.

Five months in the sisters' lives have passed when we reach the third story in the sequence, **'Panteón de Dolores'**. Sally's condition has deteriorated. She is confined to her room where even her chemo must now be delivered. The spectre of death and dark memories of their mother haunt every line. Returning to the character's name in previous stories, Dolores's thoughts and feelings about the fast-approaching loss of her sister spill out. The Mexican tradition of marking death by making a beautiful and festive *ofrenda* (offering) was embraced by Sally on her mother's death. Now, an *ofrenda* is created for Sally, with symbols of all the people and places she loved over her lifetime. The exclusion of any symbol of their mother, however unintentional, discloses just how tortuously complex and traumatising this relationship has been for both sisters. Memories flow of the sisters' peripatetic early years in a series of nondescript mining towns. The only constant is their mother's growing unhappiness and developing alcoholism, which firstly dominates and then slowly destroys their childhood. Their father's response is to continually send their mother to her room where eventually she spends most of her time. Now it is the sisters who are confined for months to Sally's bedroom in Mexico, talking and reading aloud, while Sally eagerly awaits the precious moment when sunlight enters. Dolores gives Sally the greatest gifts that a loving sister can give to a person dying of cancer – her time, loving support, and undivided attention.

> "Sally is never alone. At night I stay until I am sure she is asleep. There is no guide to death. No one to tell you what to do, how it's going to be."

Dolores's thoughts return again to their mother as she tries to understand what made her such a cruel person, filled with hate and spite. The ease and comfort of her mother's earliest years were drastically transformed by a combination of the Depression and their grandfather's alcoholism and gambling. Poverty scarred their mother, but Dolores suspects there was something else, something that damaged her irreparably. When that something is revealed, it is as shocking as it is unexpected. The gravity of Dolores's suspicion is intensified by Berlin's matter of fact delivery. As Dolores considers the mix of reasons why their mother hated Mexico so intensely, she muses about her own conflicted response to Mexico City and its culture. In so doing, her deep-seated fear of becoming like her mother rears its head yet again.

In another of Berlin's entertaining and seemingly random shifts in direction, we are told of Dolores's attempts to help Sally get everything in order, including tackling repairs to Sally's ramshackle home. The annoying but funny antics of the inept Mexican workmen tackling the repairs bring Dolores to boiling point. She finally explodes, telling them to leave as they are disturbing her gravely ill sister. The workmen respond empathetically, taking the drastic step of removing the damaged doors from their hinges to carry out repairs out of earshot. It is a touching portrayal of some of the endearing qualities at the heart of Mexican culture.

Dolores tries to care for Sally and anticipate all her needs, both physical and emotional. But dying is ultimately a solitary process and Berlin subtly reminds the reader that Sally must carry that weight alone. Our understanding of what Sally must endure is astutely linked with how their mother suffered. Another Berlin story ends with remarkable last lines as Dolores recounts a disturbing childhood memory. This time we are moved by the tears of both mother and daughter as each of them endures her solitary struggle.

If I had to pick just one Berlin story, it would certainly be the penultimate one, **'Mama'**. What Berlin has to say about dealing with terminal illness, and the turmoil it creates, is vividly portrayed in this story and her gift for balancing fear and dread with wickedly funny moments is shown to best advantage. In fact, all the hallmarks of her work are displayed here. She scrutinises pernicious mothering with empathy and tenderness. Her clear-eyed grasp of human motivation and of the terrifying capacity of parents to inflict terrible damage on their children is revealed. As the sisters attempt to fully understand their mother's actions, Berlin reminds us that the drive to come to terms with the ambiguities and complexities of human feelings and relationships is not only universal but always critical for our psychological wellbeing, most especially as death approaches.

A series of funny episodes are recalled that make the reader laugh but also get progressively darker, gradually building up a disturbing picture. While the sisters agree that their mother was undoubtedly witty, her terrible cruelty, regularly directed at her daughters, is also acknowledged. Sally laments the many ways in which her mother excluded her, yet somehow never managed to kill Sally's desperate need for maternal contact. Berlin chooses to reveal one horrifying example of their mother's callousness, when Sally travelled from Mexico following her father's death.

> "'I miss Daddy,' Sally called to her mother through the glass. 'I am dying of cancer. I need you now, Mama!' Our mother just closed the venetian blinds and ignored the banging banging on her door."

The agony of a lifetime of rejection, and her heart-breaking memories, torment Sally and give her no respite even as she is dying. Dolores finds a moving and effective way to help Sally attain longed-for peace.

> "Finally she was very sick and ready to die. She had stopped worrying about her children. She was serene, so lovely and sweet. Still, once in a while, rage grabbed her, not letting her go, denying her peace. So every night I began to tell Sally stories, like telling fairy tales … most of all I told Sally stories about how our mother once was. Before she drank, before she harmed us. Once upon a time."

Dolores's tales are peppered with explanations and justifications for their mother's actions as she works to persuade Sally that it is okay to forgive. She knows her sister well and understands her intense need to let go of a lifetime of pent-up rage and sadness. As always with Berlin, there is a final twist in the story in the very last poignant line.

This one story changed me forever. It nudged me over a threshold that I had only been dimly aware of. A determination to work hard to fully understand my own feelings and nature resulted. Lucia Berlin's stories inspired me to think deeply about my relationships with family and friends. I am a different person, and I hope a better person, because of her acuity as an observer of human behaviour.

Inevitably, the last story, **'Wait a Minute'**, brings us through the sisters' final days together. It ends years after Sally's death with a glimpse of an ageing Dolores pondering the nature of loss and grief. A strong theme running through the entire story is how our concept of time shifts, warps and oftentimes fractures under the weight of terminal cancer, the dying process, death and bereavement. The story opens with a description of what happens to time that is powerful and truthful. As only the most gifted writers can do, Berlin captures the nature of these universal experiences.

> "Time stops when someone dies. Of course it stops for them, maybe, but for the mourners time runs amok. Death comes too soon. It forgets the tides, the days growing longer and shorter, the moon. It rips up the calendar …The bad part is that when you return to your ordinary life all the routines, the marks of the day, seem like senseless lies. All is suspect, a trick to lull us, to rock us back into the placid relentlessness of time …When someone has a terminal disease, the soothing churn of time is shattered … Or time turns sadistically slow. Death just hangs around while you wait for it to be night and then wait for it to be morning. Every day you've said good-bye a little."

Dolores reflects on the stages Sally goes through as she tries to accept her fast-approaching death. We learn of moments when she weeps openly and can be comforted. More difficult are those times when she is too distraught to seek or indeed accept comfort, and so tries to muffle her tears. Hardest of all are the very last days when the weeping stops and the silence is deafening. Thankfully, humour is never far away in any Berlin story and rescues us at key points. However funny, the poignancy of these moments is not lost on the reader.

As Dolores looks back on her precious time with her sister she recalls when she first received the call from Sally to come immediately. Sally purposely gave the impression that time was short and she had at best a month to live. Dolores immediately quit her job and flew to Mexico City only to find out from Sally's oncologist on arrival that Sally was still on maintenance chemo and had at least six months to a year or perhaps more to live. Sally's explanation was truthful, affecting and as Berlin puts it, devoid of "guile or self-pity."

Berlin writes with such sweet tenderness about the sisters' mutual love and trust. We are told that over the years of remission the bond was transformed through ongoing contact and regular trips together. Now, in these last days and confined to Sally's room, the sisters sort out Sally's affairs, gossip, tell stories, and are simply present for each other. Berlin hits upon the awful reality of how, despite early promises, many disappear over the course of a terminal illness. This in turn reinforces the importance of Dolores's permanent presence by Sally's side in her dying days.

Even in the ever-darkening days of Sally's life, Berlin still finds a way to lighten things. With both her ex-husband and her lover calling to see Sally every day it falls to Dolores to ensure that they are kept apart. A farcical scene unfolds at one point when both men arrive at the same time and Dolores has to bundle the lover out of view. The reader can only smile, not only at the scene but also at what it says about Sally's attitude to the men in her life. As the end nears, Dolores moves Sally's bed closer to the window so that she can feel the sun and see the sky. Renowned as the master of the fragment, Berlin conveys so much in just a few superbly chosen words. As Dolores weeps for her sister, Sally hears and acknowledges those tears, revealing their deep, mutual love. It is yet another reminder of how carefully constructed Berlin's work is. This image of tears flowing has recurred time and again at key moments over the course of the sisters' journey together. This is the tenderest and most loving dialogue between the sisters in any of the five stories. It is no accident that Berlin has made it the very last dialogue we hear.

In a short last sequence, an ageing Dolores reflects on all the loved ones that she has lost. It is seven years since Sally died and, predictably, time has flown by. Yet Dolores also reminds us that there is never enough time. Berlin delivers another unforgettable ending, replete with an aching sense of loss.

> "I go for months without thinking of anyone but the living, and then Buddy will come with a joke, or there you vividly are, evoked by a tango or an *agua de sandia* ...You last arrived a few days after the blizzard. Ice and snow still covered the ground, but we had a fluke of a warm day ... The sun touched the teapot and the flour jar, the silver vase of stock. A lazy illumination, like a Mexican afternoon in your room. I could see the sun in your face."

Sadly, the loving and supportive sibling relationship portrayed by Berlin is not something everyone dealing with cancer can count on. Cancer literature, on the other hand, is always present, delivering meaningful human connection and providing just the right material to handle crises. There is no finer writing about the cancer experience than Lucia Berlin's. The human struggle with pain, loss, suffering and grief is superbly articulated. As the writer Lydia Davis states, it is "exhilarating writing". I can only add that it makes for exhilarating reading, helping us to endure suffering and find solace. Something magical awaits the battered soul when reading a Lucia Berlin short story. There really is no one quite like her.

'People Like That Are the Only People Here: Canonical Babbling in Peed Onk'
from *Birds of America* (1998).

First published in The New Yorker

Lorrie Moore

(*American writer. Born 1957*)

Lorrie Moore's *Birds of America* first caught my attention when it won the Irish Times International Fiction Prize in 1999. This multi-award-winning collection contains the highly regarded short story 'People Like That Are the Only People Here'. It is a story that I will never forget. My deepest maternal fears were aroused, as my own child was just a toddler then. Memories of the story resurfaced when I read Peter De Vries's novel *The Blood of the Lamb*. Though they were written close to forty years apart, the similarities between the two works are striking. De Vries's novel and Moore's short story are both howls of agonising parental fear and desperation when confronted with the unthinkable – a beloved child diagnosed with cancer. Both chose a fictional form to write about the horrifying parental impact of childhood cancer, but the reader senses the autobiographical basis underpinning their stories. De Vries and Moore also share striking comedic skills. Humour, wit and wordplay are adroitly integrated into what has to be every parent's worst nightmare.

'People Like That' can be read in two distinct and really interesting ways. Firstly, Moore articulates the lived experience of parental suffering. She reveals the immense capacity of parental love when faced with a child in mortal danger from cancer. Secondly, the process of writing about personal tragedy and the dilemmas it creates for the writer are considered. Moore achieves this dual aspect effect by making the main character – the mother – a writer. Her struggles to find a narrative route that proves true to this traumatic experience, yet also enables her to understand and endure it, are exposed. The reader cannot help but assume that the dilemmas faced reflect Moore's personal experiences.

The story begins with an unforgettable paragraph. It plunges the reader straight into a nightmarish tale of mortal threat, not only to a baby but also to a mother's sense of identity. The palpable feelings of terror and desperation set the tone for the story. Moore also establishes how the perception of time changes the moment the threat of cancer arises.

> A beginning, an end: there seems to be neither. The whole thing is like a cloud that just lands and everywhere inside it is full of rain. A start: the Mother finds a blood clot in the Baby's diaper ... what is this thing, startling against the white diaper, like a tiny mouse heart packed in snow? ... In her mind, the Mother takes this away from his body and attaches it to someone else's. There. Doesn't that make more sense?

The story moves quickly from discovery of the blood clot to attendance at the clinic in the children's hospital, where the Mother's son (the Baby) is diagnosed with a rare renal cancer. Mother, Baby and Husband find themselves thrust into the surreal world of a paediatric oncology ward (Peed Onk).

Moore withholds proper names from the main characters – the Mother, the Baby and the Husband – and refers to key hospital staff only by their titles – the Radiologist, the Surgeon, the Oncologist, the Anaesthesiologist. She even capitalises those titles to reinforce the message, conveying an unspoken truth about hospital life which is all too familiar to those living with cancer. Institutionalised hospital care reduces everyone to their role. Holding on to a sense of identity in this surreal world is a nigh on impossible task. In choosing to create an all-male line up of doctors, Moore reinforces the image of the hospital's patriarchal and hierarchical culture. It is a culture which is inappropriate and woefully inadequate for patients and carers alike. Pushing against this reality, Moore puts the Mother at the centre, telling the story from her point of view as she fiercely resists all attempts to pigeonhole her. There is no passive acceptance of what the men with power say or do. We see her constantly questioning, frustrated and angered by their failure to communicate or to connect in any meaningful way.

Moore's harrowing descriptions of the Mother's anguish are deeply moving. When she hears the Baby's diagnosis for the first time, the Mother's world collapses. A short time later, the Mother is at home, rocking the Baby to sleep while attempting to come to terms with her family's new reality. She reveals the depth and fierceness of parental love. With the Husband's arrival home, Moore jolts the reader into a consciousness of just how easily the Mother's story could be ours. She places the fragility and uncertainty of life centre stage, forcing us to consider how tragedy can befall any parent at any time. The Mother's anguished and desperate cry for a means of escape is agonising.

> What words can be uttered? You turn just slightly and there it is: the death of your child. It is part symbol, part devil, and in your blind spot all along, until, if you are unlucky, it is completely upon you. Then it is a fierce little country abducting you; it holds you squarely inside itself like a cellar room – the best boundaries of you are the boundaries of it. Are there windows? Sometimes aren't there windows?

Moore's scathing portrayal of medics devoid of empathy, lacking communication skills, and resorting to clichés, is witty and darkly humorous but also troubling. There is more than a kernel of truth in her words. The Mother satirises the usage of medical terms and derides the absurdity of the language of medics by relating it to "canonical babbling" (baby talk). Moore uncovers the bombastic nature of what passes for medical discourse and shatters the cultivated image of absolute medical authority.

She begins with a surreal conversation with the Surgeon who delivers the cancer diagnosis. This is followed by an equally surreal meeting with the Oncologist. The worst failure of empathy and sensitivity is brilliantly located by Moore at the precise moment of greatest parental fear. As the Mother and the Husband await the Surgeon's pronouncement on the outcome of the Baby's surgery and its prognostic implications, and in a room full of medical students and nurses, the Surgeon asks to speak to the Mother alone. Blithely unaware of the terror he has induced that the worst possible news is about to be delivered, he "merrily" and with a "big, spirited grin" asks the Mother to sign a copy of her book. Then, in response to her question about the condition of her Baby he responds with a throwaway comment: "The Boy? The boy is going to be fine." It is a ghastly and cringeworthy moment and one that the reader speculates might have some basis in Moore's own traumatic experience.

Medical ineptitude is revealed when the Mother spots that something has gone awry following the Baby's surgery. A nurse is called and is quickly followed by a medical student. The gallows humour of what follows is deeply unsettling.

> Valerie is a saint, but her voice is the standard hospital saint voice: an infuriating, pharmaceutical calm. It says, Everything is normal here. Death is normal. Pain is normal. Nothing is abnormal … the attending physician is a medical student. He looks fifteen. The authority he attempts to convey, he cannot remotely inhabit.

Finally, the Mother succeeds in getting the matter resolved but concludes:

> And still, and still: look at all the things you have to do to protect a child, a hospital merely an intensification of life's cruel obstacle course.

Moore reminds the reader of just how crucial patient advocacy is in the hospital environment. It is a harsh reality that cancer patients and carers encounter daily.

Moore's perspective on the community of parents – the 'People Like That' of the title who populate Peed Onk and the Tiny Tim Lounge for parents – is refreshingly different from many childhood cancer narratives, both fictional and autobiographical. Interesting parallels can be found with how Peter De Vries portrays that same community in *The Blood of the Lamb*. Whilst the Husband in Moore's book takes comfort in being with fellow sufferers, throwing himself into that community and sharing stories, the Mother fiercely resists, distancing herself at every turn. She is irritated by the Husband's response as she herself can find no solace in that world. The survival of her identity and that of her family is tied to a fierce resistance to becoming part of such a community or accepting such a fate. Escaping from the world of Peed Onk and the Tiny Tim Lounge is the only tolerable option. The Mother confirms that life would be meaningless without the Baby and so she would choose suicide rather than join that community and watch her child die. For the Mother, it is normal life or no life at all.

'People Like That' reads like a story that had to be told. Utterly believable, it shines a light on deeply painful aspects of the cancer experience. Truths about life's fragility and our ever-present human vulnerability to potential tragedy are chillingly told. It is an unforgettable cancer story and a powerful reminder of the power of fiction in helping us process traumatic experiences.

'I Want to Live!'
from *The Pugilist at Rest* (1993).
First published in Harper's Magazine

Thom Jones
(American writer 1945–2016)

I somehow missed Thom Jones's meteoric arrival onto the literary scene in the early 1990s. Although 'I Want to Live!' has been widely anthologised and critically lauded, I must confess that it had escaped my attention. I had dipped into John Updike's *The Best American Short Stories of the Century*, but never landed on Jones's story until research pointed me in that direction. What a discovery. It reminds me at every turn of Tolstoy's novella *The Death of Ivan Ilyich*.

'I Want to Live!' is a perfectly formed short story with a narrative drive that grabs hold of the reader from the first paragraph and never eases its grip. Jones mirrors key themes of Tolstoy's work, themes that are central concerns for people living with cancer. The physical and psychological journey through cancer hell is presented in explicit and unflinching detail. The fear of approaching death and the impulse it engenders to reflect on a previously unexamined life is explored. Jones probes the wisdom that sometimes comes from grappling with suffering. The true nature of family life and of friendship is revealed together with the critical importance of empathetic care when dealing with horrific pain and suffering. Overarching it all is a touching account of human resilience and the desire to live at all costs. Jones's short story encompasses all of these themes. It is a riveting and darkly humorous portrait of a woman's inexorable descent through terminal cancer and on to death.

The gritty realism of Jones's portrayal of the dying process – from diagnosis, through surgery, chemotherapy cycles, a brief respite, and then swift decline – is raw and convincing. His no-holds-barred approach leaves us in no doubt about the physical pain and psychological suffering experienced by Mrs Wilson, an ordinary woman with advanced cancer. That awful moment of first hearing a cancer diagnosis is brilliantly depicted.

> She looked past the thin oncologist, wire-rimmed glasses, white coat, inscrutable. Outside, snowflakes tumbled from the sky, kissing the pavement – each unique, wonderful, worth an hour of study, a microcosm of the Whole: awe-inspiring, absolutely fascinating, a gift of divinity gratis. Yet how abhorrent they seemed. They were white, but the whole world had lost its color for her now that she'd heard those words. The shine was gone from the world. Had she been Queen of the Universe for a million years and witnessed glory after glory, what would it have mattered now that she had come to this?

Mrs Wilson's fortitude and resilience emerge as she undergoes the intensifying horrors of fifteen cycles of chemotherapy. The only modicum of relief for the reader comes from the welcome touches of grim humour woven through her monologue. It is writing charged not only with physical pain but also with psychological suffering. At first, Mrs Wilson wonders what became of her childhood hopes and expectations. The realisation of what her life has been, and the feeling that she has never really lived, haunt her. Yet her furious will to survive treatment and live again is never in question. Anger raises its head and the nights spent alone become unbearable. Her oncologist's lack of empathy is writ large throughout. It is an object lesson in how patients can be utterly failed by those tasked with their care.

> The whole problem with him was that he didn't seem real. He wasn't a flesh-and-blood kinda guy. Where was the *empathy*? Why did he get into this field if he couldn't empathize? In this field, empathy should be your stock-in-trade.

Relief finally arrives from the most unexpected source. It is her son-in-law who proves to be her saviour. His capacity for empathy ensures that his presence alone provides indispensable support. The son-in-law's interventions, practical and psychological, come precisely at her moments of greatest need. As her condition deteriorates, her physical pain worsens, and is poorly managed by her doctor. With his encyclopaedic knowledge of prescription drugs, her son-in-law successfully advocates on her behalf, absolutely determined to relieve her suffering.

As Mrs Wilson's body declines, her psychological struggles grow ever more pressing, threatening to overwhelm her. Thoughts of death, the desperate need to make sense of her life and her troubled relationship with her daughter all prove distressing. It is her son-in-law who helps her to find a way through this morass of growing mental anguish. He introduces Mrs Wilson to Schopenhauer's philosophy. Insights flow from her reading of Schopenhauer and from lively and laughter-filled philosophical discussions with her son-in-law. The value of truth and of laughter become apparent to her as she delves into Schopenhauer's pessimistic vision. It brings solace, despite her growing physical pain.

> Yet Schopenhauer got right into the heart of all the important things. The things that really mattered. With Schopenhauer she could take long excursions from the grim specter of impending death. In Schopenhauer, particularly in his aphorisms and reflections, she found an absolute satisfaction, for Schopenhauer spoke the truth and the rest of the world was disseminating lies!

There is a touching, if brief, period of respite when she returns to her home and sees her friends. The insight she has gained into matters of life and death sharpens her perceptions.

In a richly comedic and surreal twist, Jones chooses to tease out Schopenhauer's philosophy by introducing a bantam red rooster named Mr Barnes to the story. As death draws ever closer, Mrs Wilson's overwhelming desire to live is paramount. Her mind wanders in a haze of morphine sulphate and she remembers a much-loved little red rooster at the farm where she grew up. She concludes that he was the very personification of Schopenhauer's concept of the Will to Live and had she been more like him she might have pursued her dreams and so achieved a more meaningful and worthwhile life.

> That Barnes – he was something. She should have taken a lesson.

Puffed out her chest and walked through life – "I want the biggest and the best and the most of whatever you've got!" There were people who pulled it off. You really could do it if you had the attitude.

Jones's realistic representation of Mrs Wilson's death is gripping. Her last thoughts are of love and of the words that she has left unsaid. As with other chosen stories, there is a real sense in 'I Want to Live!' of autobiography and fiction conflating. The mirroring of Tolstoy's work is a powerful reminder of how cancer literature's rich legacy inspires new writing. Regardless of where Jones drew inspiration from, he has managed to create something altogether new, fresh and vital. There is honesty and emotional power in a story delivered through a superb monologue, vivid characters, and grimly comedic touches. In less skilful hands, this portrait of human suffering could have been a depressing read. In Jones's hands, 'I Want to Live!' is uplifting and brimming with empathy, wisdom, resilience and humanity.

'Floating Bridge'
from *Hateship, Friendship, Courtship, Loveship, Marriage* (2001)

First published in The New Yorker

Alice Munro

(Canadian writer. Born 1931)

There was never any doubt that Munro, the master of the short story form and a long-time personal favourite, would appear in this collection. Many Munro stories deal with the subject of cancer but one in particular eclipsed all others for me. 'Floating Bridge' is a triumph. The universality of the central character's inner turmoil connects with the reader at a gut level. As always with Munro, we are instantly sucked into the raging undercurrents in the mind of the story's central character. This beautifully balanced short story is a powerful meditation on mortality and on the psychological challenges and complexities of living at the edge of life and death.

   Key features and themes for which Munro is loved and lauded in equal measure are present. It is the story of Jinny, an ordinary woman shaped by choices and compromises made over a lifetime. When we meet her, a moment of crisis has arrived that abruptly shifts her perspective and forces her to confront issues that she has long been ignoring. Trapped in an unsatisfying relationship that seems devoid of real connection, she is also in danger of losing her sense of identity. Over the course of one day and an eventful journey, both psychological and physical, Jinny reflects on her life. Shuttling back and forth in time and memory, she searches for self-understanding. Unpredictable shifts in point of view occur as the story progresses. The complex nature of one woman's inner life is ever so delicately laid bare. Munro's trademark ambiguous and non-judgemental approach offers no clear-cut resolutions. Instead, the reader is drawn into considering alternative interpretations of the jumble of psychological and emotional issues flooding Jinny's mind.

As one would expect from Munro, cancer is woven into the fabric of the story in a richly imaginative and unique way. When we first meet Jinny, she is leaving the hospital following an appointment with an oncologist. She is deeply unsettled by news about her disease, but that news is not shared with the reader until much later on in the narrative.

> The parked cars, the pavement, the bricks of the other buildings, seemed positively to bombard her, as if they were all separate facts thrown up in ridiculous sequence. She did not take changes of scene very well these days, she wanted everything familiar and stable. It was the same with changes of information.

Jinny's unsatisfactory relationship with her partner, Neal, and his lightweight nature are swiftly established. As Neal picks Jinny up, he asks no questions about her appointment. His focus is instead on Helen, the girl waiting in their van whom he has hired as home help for the expected last stages of Jinny's terminal cancer. Jinny chooses to remain silent. Her one tentative attempt to broach her medical news arises when she is briefly alone with Neal but he is deaf to her concerns, not only distracted but fecklessly detached. The journey home commences but proves circuitous in a myriad of ways.

It is apparent that Jinny has come to terms with her imminent death and taken it as licence to ignore all that is wrong with her life. This abdication of personal responsibility is linked with the dramatic change of perception wrought by terminal cancer. Matters that she had agonised over in her life before cancer are now seen as trivial and of little account. For Jinny, cancer has, ironically, been a liberation of sorts. Her will to live is questionable.

> And yet – an excitement. The unspeakable excitement you feel when a galloping disaster promises to release you from all responsibility for your own life.

As the story progresses, Munro continues to withhold the oncologist's latest news. Remission is suggested, however, by the fact that Jinny's emotions have been thrown out of kilter. Her sense of freedom has suddenly evaporated and she has been hurled back into a world of uncertainty. The distress that test results, whether they are ostensibly good or bad, often generate in the cancer patient is perfectly captured. Jinny's physical discomfort, anxiety and sense of dislocation build as Neal diverts from the direct route home. On a spurious errand, he drives through street scenes that are bleak and depressing. Arriving at a trailer home, Neal is determined to accept an invitation from the owners, June and Matt, to visit, seemingly oblivious to Jinny's needs and her fragile state. Left alone in the van, Jinny considers the real nature of Neal's interest in Helen. There is a suggestion that Neal may previously have had affairs that she chose to ignore. In growing physical and emotional discomfort, Jinny leaves the van and seeks relief and shade in a nearby cornfield. It is as if the medical news has released her suppressed anger not only at Neal but also at herself for staying silent and not addressing her flawed relationship. Munro provides a wonderful analogy for Jinny's mounting psychological and emotional distress in her description of Jinny's panic when she gets lost in the cornfield.

> She had stepped over one row and then another and probably got turned around. She tried going back the way she had come, but it obviously wasn't the right way. There were clouds over the sun again so she couldn't tell where she was. And she had not known which direction she was going when she entered the field, so that would not have helped anyway ... Her heart was pounding just like any heart that had years and years of life ahead of it.

Barking dogs and Matt's voice lead her out of the cornfield and back to the van. As Matt tells a coarse joke, Jinny is consumed by anxiety and so hears none of it. Instead, the words of her oncologist come back to her and the reader finally learns what has transpired.

> "I do not wish to give the wrong impression. We must not get carried away with optimism. But it looks as if we have some unexpected results here ... It looks as if there has been very significant shrinkage. What we hoped for of course but frankly we did not expect it. And I do not mean that the battle is over, just that it is a favorable sign ...

Quite a favorable sign. We do not know that there may not be more trouble in the future but we can say we are cautiously optimistic."

This stay of execution – a reprieve of sorts – offers hope, but it is a hope that is hedged all around with uncertainty. Hard days of further treatment may lie ahead. The dying process may have been simply extended. Yet recovery is now also a possibility that has to be considered. Having shed all hope and accepted impending death, for Jinny this turnaround is as difficult as it is unexpected. It also means that, with remission, her deep concerns about the nuts and bolts of her life can no longer be ignored. As always with Munro there is a huge amount to be inferred. The rush of thoughts and feelings, building up since the start of the story, becomes almost unbearable.

A new character arrives into the story at this point. Ricky is a young man of whom Jinny knows nothing yet he provides the first glimmer of understanding and compassion to appear in the story. His empathy is in marked contrast to Neal's behaviour.

> He seemed to understand things, though. He seemed to understand that she was exhausted and in some kind of a muddle.

Ricky offers to drive her home when she refuses to let him call on Neal to do so. As the journey home begins, Ricky takes a deserted road, blithely informing Jinny that there is no danger of meeting anybody and explaining that he won't turn the car lights on until they can see the stars. There is a feeling that Jinny is stepping out of time, escaping her normal life and moving towards an experience that could prove risky. The ominous tone builds as the journey continues. Jinny soon realises that the road is surrounded by water and Ricky informs her that they are crossing a swamp. Stopping the van, he instructs her to get out and walk with him. He leads her to a floating bridge and insists she walks out onto it. It is a moment Munro imbues with the magic and mystery of the natural world and the world of the mind.

> The slight movement of the bridge made her imagine that all the trees and the reed beds were set on saucers of earth and the road was a floating ribbon of earth and underneath it all was water. And the water seemed so still, but it could not really be still because if you tried to keep your eye on one reflected star, you saw how it winked

and changed shape and slid from sight. Then it was back again – but maybe not the same one.

The magic is amplified precisely because it is a shared moment of real human connection. Jinny suddenly realises that she has been without her hat since meeting Ricky so her bald head has been exposed and yet it has not mattered. It is a moment of epiphany for Jinny as she loses all sense of unease and accepts the uncertain ground that she is on. She realises that this chance encounter, together with her willingness to take a risk, has generated an experience that is breathtakingly honest and true. The moment ends with a shared kiss.

As is Munro's style, the story has a deliberately ambiguous ending. Jinny thinks of and feels compassion for Neal, "back on dry land" and considering his future. She herself has at last found peace in her inner world and for now that is enough.

One over-arching concern lies at the root of Jinny's turmoil and it is one that readers living and dying with cancer know all too well. Given how precious life is, how do we come to terms with our mortality? How do we find a way to acknowledge it? How do we accept life's precariousness and unpredictability and still live meaningfully and fully, true to who we are? The floating bridge is an inspired metaphor for Jinny's moment of epiphany, shattering the illusion that solid ground exists for anyone in life and reminding us that forever shifting and insecure ground is our only reality. Arguably, the threat to Jinny lies as much in the possibility of loss of self as it does in cancer. Jinny's moment of clarity suggests that, however precarious, this unsteady ground and this self are all that we can count on. And yet, they are also all that we need to sustain a meaningful existence. It is an empowering, empathetic and deeply consoling message for the reader.

'Light'
from *Olive, Again* (2019)

Elizabeth Strout

(American writer. Born 1956)

Now and then a perfectly realised fictional character comes along that takes hold of the reader's imagination and lodges there. Olive Kitteridge is one such rare character, remarkable and unforgettable. She first appeared in Elizabeth Strout's 2008 Pulitzer prize-winning book *Olive Kitteridge*. In a collection of 13 interconnected short stories, Strout created a luminous portrait of provincial life in a coastal town in Maine. Skilfully peeling back the layers of small-town life, she revealed the loneliness, quiet desperation, petty prejudices, trauma and devastation that lie beneath a seemingly tranquil and mundane surface. Olive is a vivid and vital presence at the heart of Strout's book, whether playing a central role in some stories or just a minor part in others. A flavour of her contrary personality is captured beautifully in just two sentences.

> She didn't like to be alone. Even more, she didn't like being with people.

With every appearance, Strout slowly builds our understanding of this indomitable character as she struggles to know herself and the people around her. This flawed woman, who is never less than brutally honest with herself and others, has wormed her way into our hearts by the book's end. She is at times difficult, stubborn, brusque, grumpy, infuriating and socially inept. And yet she is also vulnerable, insightful, intuitive and empathetic. Perhaps her most endearing characteristic is her instinctive compassion for those in crisis and desperately in need of kindness and support. When a sequel finally appeared it contained a powerful story that might have been tailor-made for this collection.

In the story 'Light,' Strout gives a deeply affecting and multifaceted portrait of a cancer patient. At first glance, Cindy Coombs seems to be an ordinary woman shaped by a childhood of poverty and struggle. By dint of hard work she has created a good life. Happily married and with two sons at university, she worked as a librarian until diagnosed with cancer. She is a woman with a reflective nature, a poet's soul, and a deep love of literature. Strout reveals Cindy's poetic sensibility in a beautiful passage as Cindy recuperates from chemotherapy and considers the light in February, relishing the promise it holds.

> ... for Cindy the light of the month had always been like a secret, and it remained a secret even now ... You could see how at the end of each day the world seemed cracked open and the extra light made its way across the stark trees, and promised. It *promised*, that light, and what a thing that was. As Cindy lay on her bed she could see this even now, the gold of the last light opening the world.

When we first meet Cindy, she is nearing the end of a series of chemotherapy cycles. Under gentle, well-meaning but ill-considered pressure from her husband, Tom, she reluctantly ventures out to the local supermarket. Physically and emotionally unprepared, Cindy is quickly overwhelmed. Luckily, rescue is at hand in the shape of her former teacher, Olive Kitteridge. Sensing the depth of Cindy's distress, Olive follows up the chance meeting with three unsolicited visits to Cindy's home. What unfolds over these three short visits is a touching portrayal of the transformative power of human connection.

Cindy is grateful when Olive arrives unexpectedly for the first visit. She is moved by the affinity she feels for this former teacher whom she hardly knows. She senses that Olive is a woman with the capacity not only to listen but also to understand what she is going through. Olive's customary forthright and honest approach enables Cindy to open up and talk about the frustrations and emotions which have been building up for months. Presented at last with a meaningful opportunity to talk about her feelings, Cindy reveals her loneliness, her sense of isolation, her anger and her fear of death. Olive in turn divulges the deep regret she feels about failing her first husband in his last years. In Strout's beautifully controlled rendering, their intimate dialogue unfolds naturally and believably. Both women gain insight and find comfort in each other. Olive's final words of reassurance as this first visit comes to an end are a testimony to a universal truth and exactly what Cindy has needed to hear.

> They were quiet. Cindy felt – she almost felt normal. "Well," she said finally. "It's just that I'm so alone. I don't want to be so alone."
> "Course you don't."
> "You're scared to die, even at your age?"
> Olive nodded … Then Olive said, "You know, Cindy, if you *should* be dying, if you do die, the truth is – we're all just a few steps behind you. Twenty minutes behind you, and that's the truth."
> Cindy had not thought of that … But Olive was right: They were all headed where she was going. If she was going.
> "Thank you," Cindy said. "And thank you for coming over."

The emotional honesty that marked Olive's first visit resumes on her second. Further intimate revelations flow between the women. Cindy's deep concerns will be all too familiar to cancer patients. Although she has the support of one stalwart friend – her sister-in-law Anita – she is profoundly upset and at a loss to understand why old friends have deserted her. She expresses her deep-seated fear of leaving her husband alone should she die, yet paradoxically how the thought of him being with someone else breaks her heart. Olive consoles her from the standpoint of her personal experience. She tells Cindy how her love for her first husband is as strong as ever, as is her grief and sense of loss, even as she continues on living a full life with her second husband.

> "I'm awfully glad you come over," Cindy said. "You wouldn't believe the people who don't come over to see me."
> "Yes, I would. Believe it."
> "But why don't they come to see me? I mean, Olive. Old *friends* don't even come to see me."
> "They're scared."
> "Well, too bad!"
> "Oh, I agree. I agree with you about that."
> "But you're not scared."
> "Nope."

"Even though you're scared of dying."
"That's right," Olive said.

Olive's third visit comes just a week after Cindy's final treatment and in that difficult waiting period before the three-month scan to see if chemotherapy has worked. As they share further confidences it is clear that both women have created an unexpected and transformative connection at a critical moment in their lives. Being able to articulate their deepest concerns and reveal their wounds to someone who comprehends them helps alleviate their loneliness and isolation. Strout avoids the resolution that we might expect if this were a novel, namely explicitly disclosing whether Cindy lives or dies. By so doing she enables the focus to remain on the significance of what has happened between Cindy and Olive. The story ends with a wonderfully transcendent moment, full of the joy and hope that flows from meaningful human connection and from unexpectedly finding a kindred spirit. Bravo Elizabeth Strout!

> "Would you look at that," Olive said. Cindy turned to look. The sunlight was magnificent, it shone a glorious yellow from the pale blue sky, and through the bare branches of the trees, with the open-throated look that came toward the end of the day's light. But here is what happened next – Here is the thing that Cindy, for the rest of her life, would never forget: Olive Kitteridge said, "My god, but I have always loved the light in February." Olive shook her head slowly. "My God," she repeated, with awe in her voice. "Just look at that February light."

'Tell Me a Riddle'
from *Tell Me a Riddle* (1961).
First published in New World Writing

Tillie Olsen
(American writer 1912–2007)

The sweetest discovery of my first year working as a librarian was a series of books produced by a new arrival to the publishing world. The Virago Modern Classics, with their distinctive green spines and apple logo, celebrated women's experiences. A diverse range of literary female voices from different generations and cultures were finally brought together. For some, Virago was their first publisher, whilst others had been neglected or long forgotten. If a book made it onto this fledgling list, quality was assured. I became a dedicated follower, eagerly awaiting new titles. Virago cracked open and then reshaped my reading experience at a formative time. It is where I first encountered Tillie Olsen's story 'Tell Me a Riddle'. Beautifully crafted and thematically rich, this revered classic touches on issues of gender, class and social justice. I grew up in a society where the evidence of women's lives utterly constrained by poverty, motherhood and societal expectations was all around me. Sadly, it took Olsen's story to truly open my eyes to the tragic consequences. 'Tell Me a Riddle' uncovers how such forces stunt one woman's life and, in consequence, stealthily destroy her marriage and her family relationships. This loving family, already living in a fog of misunderstanding, is driven into crisis when it is suddenly forced to deal with a terminal cancer diagnosis.

Olsen depicts the inner life of a disillusioned and ageing woman with cancer who is weighed down by a lifetime of bitter resentment and rage. Eva is struggling to find meaning and is working to rediscover her sense of self as death approaches. Her life has been severely reduced by poverty, motherhood and a patriarchal world. It is not just a woman's inner world that is set forth, however. Using multiple voices, Olsen creates a well-rounded and complex picture of a family in crisis. She probes the perspectives of wife, husband, children and finally a granddaughter as the story unfolds. The mounting disappointments and misunderstandings that escalate marital conflict and drive couples apart are exposed. It is a story full of lament for lost human potential and unfulfilled lives. It is also a moving portrayal of how the dying process can bring a measure of acceptance and a rediscovery of the self. This, in turn, makes meaningful reconnection with loved ones possible. Olsen's opening lines seize our attention and draw us straight into the story.

> For forty-seven years they had been married. How deep back the stubborn, gnarled roots of the quarrel reached, no one could say – but only now, when tending to the needs of others no longer shackled them together, the roots swelled up visible, split the earth between them, and the tearing shook even to the children, long since grown.

The central characters of Eva and David, unnamed for much of the story, are a couple who have lived marginalised and impoverished lives. Russian immigrants with a revolutionary past, they have struggled to raise seven children and, in the process, have become trapped in stereotypical roles. Their lives have been blighted by the force to conform to societal expectations. The idealistic dreams of their youth have been sacrificed and their memories of those dreams, long repressed, are now largely forgotten. Resentment and bitterness are tearing them apart in their twilight years. With the children grown, David is determined to sell their home and move to a retirement community. Eva fiercely resists. As the bickering grows and both become entrenched, hints that Eva is in poor health appear.

> She did not know if the tumult was outside, or in her. Always a ravening inside, a pull to the bed, to lie down, to succumb.

With a growing sense of unease, Eva retreats further into solitude and begins to journey back in her mind to her idealistic youth in Russia. Meanwhile, David works to bring his children on board in an effort to break down Eva's resistance. Olsen brilliantly captures the family dynamic as the adult children struggle to deal with parents who are fiercely opposed to each other. The first section of the story ends when the children learn that Eva, who has undergone gallbladder surgery, has terminal cancer.

With what they believe to be Eva's best interests at heart, father and children withhold the truth of her illness. This damaging silence is compounded by their failure to listen to Eva's desperate pleas to return home. She is effectively infantilised, kept voiceless and denied the dignity of determining for herself how to live out her remaining days. Instead, she is dragged across the country, from one adult child to another, which affords her none of the solitude that she yearns for. Eva responds in the only way open to her. She retreats further into silence and memory and refuses to engage in the ways expected of her by her grieving family. Her husband and children struggle but fail to hear or understand, and yet yearn for connection. It is a superbly nuanced and painfully moving study of family distress. As the story builds, the riddle of motherhood is scrutinised as an enriching and a destructive force. A heavy price is paid for overwhelming maternal love.

When Eva and David begin what turns out to be the last leg of their journey, a pivotal moment in the story is reached. Eva's health is rapidly deteriorating as they arrive in Los Angeles to stay in a small apartment, cared for and supported by their granddaughter, Jeannie. Finally, Eva is with a family member who intuitively understands her.

> ... the lightness and brightness of her like a healing.

Olsen uses a stream of consciousness technique that brings the reader right into Eva's mind as her retreat into memory begins to transform her. Sparked by encounters with relatives and an old friend, the clash between the materialism of her present world and the idealism of her youth comes to a head at a concert. Deeply distressed by her arduous quest for meaning and her feelings of alienation, she turns to her husband.

> And looking for an answer – in the helpless pity and fear for her (for *her*) that distorted his face – she understood the last months, and knew that she was dying.

The veil of lies is torn away, and the truth is compassionately if unintentionally revealed. As the final part of the story begins, Eva acquiesces to the continuing silence.

> She saw the fiction was necessary to him, was silent ...

Yet again her plea to return home falls on deaf ears. After a lifetime of silences, Eva enters the final days of the dying process speaking incessantly. Her repressed voice is at last released. The intensity of Eva's dying days and the conflicted responses of a loving but largely unknowing family is skilfully portrayed. For David, tenderness and compassion vie with a desire to flee from witnessing Eva's physical agonies.

> And he, who had once dreaded a long dying (from fear of himself, from horror of the dwindling money) now desired her quick death profoundly, for *her* sake.

Slowly, Eva's voice pierces the wall of silence that has separated David not only from his wife, but also from their shared idealism and his sense of self. It is a moment of epiphany.

The children arrive, one by one, to say goodbye to a mother whom they have never really understood. Nor have they known of her idealistic dreams. Now it is too late. Hope for a better future lies with Jeannie, who listens, hears and cherishes this time with Eva. Eva's quest for meaning is over and her sense of self integrity has been restored. However difficult witnessing her death-bed agonies is for her family, Eva herself is insulated from them.

> Jeannie came to comfort him. In her light voice she said: Grandaddy, Grandaddy don't cry. She is not there, she promised me. On the last day, she said she would go back to when she first heard music, a little girl on the road to the village where she was born. She promised me ... Leave her there, Grandaddy, it is all right. She promised me. Come back, come back and help her poor body to die.

'Tell Me a Riddle' has lost none of its relevance or emotional power. Olsen's story is a damning critique of the social and cultural forces that can damage individuals and prevent them from reaching their potential, with drastic consequences for families and for wider society. Olsen's vision of a socially just world that empowers individuals and transforms society is like a steady light embedded in the story's soul. It is a vision that Olsen herself vehemently believed in and struggled for. Sadly, her powerful message about the silencing of women and the erosion of women's sense of identity remains as relevant as ever, more than sixty years after her story first appeared. The theme of social justice is never allowed to obscure or overpower the story, however. Olsen's razor-sharp focus is always on her characters and their plight. Her tale reminds us that kindness, tenderness and compassion can survive the onslaught of marginalisation and alienation and can break through the silences that develop in families as a result. Not one false note is struck in this haunting portrayal of the complexities of inner lives and relationships when a loved one is faced with cancer and approaching death.

Olsen's story is a wonderful example of the timelessness, resonance and compressed power of classic short stories and novellas. I must admit it is also really gratifying to include a novella by a writer who was an avid library user. Olsen passionately believed in the power of public libraries to change lives. How right she was.

'Muriel Scaife'
from *Union Street* (1982)

Pat Barker
(English writer. Born 1943)

For the passionate reader, there is such pleasure in discovering an exceptional writer early in their writing career. Following that thrill of discovery, subsequent publications are eagerly awaited, as the reader knows with absolute certainty that this is a writer whose career should skyrocket. When it does, there is a feeling of personal satisfaction in having spotted that talent early. For me, Pat Barker is one such writer. Her first two novels were roundly rejected. It took her ten years to find a publisher for what became her debut work, *Union Street*. Regard for her work grew with every new publication and admiring reviews appeared with ever-increasing frequency. The Booker prize winning Regeneration trilogy finally brought widespread recognition and respect. As much as I have enjoyed her body of work, *Union Street* holds a special place in my heart. Classified as a novel, it is in fact a series of interconnected short stories, one of which powerfully articulates the impact of cancer and loss on one marginalised woman and her family.

It is no accident that Barker follows Olsen in this collection. Although markedly different in writing style and in socio-political and economic contexts, striking similarities exist in their work. Stinging critiques of social and economic forces that devastate individual lives and communities are presented by both writers. Feminist values lie at their core. They give voice to women rendered voiceless and forced by class and gender inequalities to live marginalised and impoverished lives. Women's experiences previously dismissed as irrelevant and unimportant are placed centre stage. Women's feelings about marital relations, sexuality, mothering, homelife and community life are interrogated. Complex stories of women's lives are constructed and presented with bleak social realism but are also highly symbolic. Barker and Olsen create narratives that, although harrowing, exhibit the strength, humour and resilience of vibrantly real characters. Of central importance to this collection is Barker's brutally honest yet delicately nuanced short story about the fragility of human life and the impact of cancer and grief on a loving family.

Muriel Scaife is one of the women living on Union Street in the 1970s whose Northern English working-class culture is declining precipitously. Barker brilliantly establishes and then builds the feeling that her characters are living in a battle zone. The now empty steelworks and the rubble of surrounding streets undergoing demolition dominate the book's physical and psychological landscape. The houses on Union Street, too, are disintegrating. Crumbling and broken, with boarded up windows, collapsing floors, and stairs and fireplaces that leak smoke and grime, these homes are as fragile as their vulnerable inhabitants. Everyone living on Union Street is struggling to survive unrelenting hardship and disempowerment in what is fast becoming a wasteland. Post-industrial dereliction is threatening to erase the last vestiges of a sustaining and sustainable community. The men of Union Street are rendered impotent and powerless by unemployment, with repercussions for every aspect of their lives. They are largely absent from home and have dysfunctional, oftentimes abusive relationships with women. Although traces of sporadic community support are still discernible, it is a community that is at best ambivalent but is also rapidly fragmenting. Each woman finds herself essentially alone and without even the possibility of self-determination. Children are particularly vulnerable and are devoid of security and sanctuary. They seem destined to follow their parents into marginalised lives in a world where any semblance of community may have disappeared. There is an oppressive atmosphere of entrapment overlying all. Barker immerses the reader in this dark place through the female perspective. It is a world that is desolate and depressing. Yet in Barker's skilful hands it is also a world tinged with the possibility of recovery and regeneration.

The structure of *Union Street* resembles that of Joyce's *Dubliners*. Each of the seven short stories is focused on the experiences of an individual woman facing a traumatic, life-changing moment. These individual stories can together be taken to symbolise the progress of one working-class woman moving through life, from childhood to old age and onto death. The story of 'Muriel Scaife', situated at the exact midpoint of the book, perfectly encapsulates all of the themes previously explored. As a standalone short story about one woman and her family enduring the trauma of cancer and loss it is exceptional.

Barker gives voice not only to Muriel's inner life but also to that of John, her dying husband, and their twelve-year-old son, Richard. This multi-voicing technique combines effectively with Barker's use of colloquial dialogue to draw us right into the heart of this family. It also enables us to fully understand the complexities of family relationships and the precarious and fragile nature of life on Union Street for every individual Scaife.

> The house was peaceful all around her, full of firelight and sleeping children … Yet, beneath the surface of her mind, something that could not be so easily lulled roused itself to keep watch … She must always be aware of time passing, of the worm that hides in darkness and feeds upon innocence, beauty and grace. John's hands on her breasts, the children asleep upstairs: nothing was to be taken for granted. Love, security, order: those were achievements painfully wrested from a chaos that was always threatening to take them back … In a moment, she told herself, she would get up and turn the telly on. The room would be full of flickering light, there would be no more pressure of darkness, no more sense that life is threatened, no more feeling that you must stay awake to guard it.

The agonising impact of cancer and death on individual family members and on the family dynamic are delicately laid bare. There is an emotional depth to the story that is deeply moving. The reader is right there with Muriel, John, and Richard, witnessing the physical horrors of advanced cancer as it destroys John's body. Barker holds nothing back in describing that physical horror and so makes the emotional and psychological toll palpably real. Barker is known for reusing images across her body of work. It is one such image that proves profoundly disturbing and compelling.

> She ran back into the living-room and there was John, blood gargling from his mouth. Above the black hole his eyes rolled about, frenzied

and unseeing ... He was choking on the blood. She began pulling huge clots of it from his mouth ... Her fingers found a thick rope of blood, twirled around it, and pulled. The clot slid out of his mouth, with the sound of a sink coming unblocked ...

Poverty and marginalisation intensify and deepen the pressure-cooker atmosphere that Muriel's family have to endure. Medical care is perfunctory. Muriel is forced by economic necessity to leave her husband even in his dying days for her school cleaning job. The depth of shared love between Muriel and John is poignantly conveyed in two beautiful images.

John slept – if he slept at all – in the armchair, with Muriel's coat over him. She had offered him an eiderdown, which would have been warmer, but no, he wanted the coat.

Muriel lay on the sofa. It was made of leather, cracked in some places, rubbed thin in others, and had not been new even when they bought it. They had made love on this sofa when they were a young married couple ... And she'd lain there in the early stages of labour ... It had seen so much of her married life. While she lay on it, nothing terrible could become real.

Concern for his family is uppermost in John's mind as death approaches. After a night when the reality of approaching death can no longer be ignored, John voices that reality.

John's eyes had closed again. After a while, they flickered open. "You'll be all right you know, Muriel. There'll be a pension. And if ever you wanted owt you'd only have to ask our Betty."

Richard, academically bright and focused on schoolwork, is perplexed by his father's hatred of books. His relationship with his father is blighted not only by John's illiteracy but also by the secrecy and shame that surrounds it. This terrible secret hinders father's and son's awkward attempts to bridge the yawning gap between them before it is too late.

What he wanted was to meet the boy on common ground: to share jokes and interests, to introduce him to the world of work, pub, football. But he couldn't do it. Of course the boy was too young, but that was the least of it. His feet were set on a different path.

Close friendships in the community that would help alleviate trauma and provide meaningful support for father, mother and son are conspicuous by their absence. Humour is introduced in the shape of Muriel's disapproving mother and Muriel's sister-in-law, Betty. It is through Betty's voice that we learn that John has Hodgkin lymphoma. Muriel's mother is introduced right at the start, signalling her important role not only within the family but also in providing the wit and laughter so desperately needed in such a bleak story.

> The bus arrived at last. Those getting on jostled those getting off and from the confusion an elderly woman emerged wearing a maroon-coloured raincoat and a professionally-martyred expression."

This totally believable character despises her son-in-law for failing to provide for his family and is dismissive of John and Muriel's tangible love. Given her own experience of poverty and her legitimate fears for her daughter, we sympathise with her standpoint. Her interventions come at key moments in the story and her presence works to great effect. When John is brought home in his coffin, her reaction lightens a little the darkness that has enveloped the family. After the funeral, she continues to behave reassuringly to type.

> The old lady's conviction that her son-in-law had enjoyed excellent health, though a little shaken by his death, was by no means overcome.

Following John's death, Muriel's shock, numbness and disbelief soon give way to overwhelming grief and despair. It is a truthful and utterly unsentimental representation of loss that is also achingly personal. Early and tentative steps towards recovery are discernible by the story's end. Mother and son are united by grief, love and growing understanding. The story closes on a hopeful note. We see a family that has every chance of surviving this huge loss and perhaps even of thriving. That glimmer of hope rests on Muriel's resilience which is already showing signs of recovery. Barker's last words suggest that Muriel is strong enough to overcome the hard times that inevitably lie ahead.

The final wonderful image is of Muriel choosing to turn away from a mirror to look instead at a magnificent moon. It gives the reader hope that it is not the careworn, grieving mother, with heavy responsibilities and a precarious future, that Muriel sees. Rather, it is her inner power and strength that is in her mind's eye, together with the possibility that life holds hope for her own and her family's future. The character of Muriel is such a skilful creation that we are invested emotionally in her story. She is no victim of circumstance or stereotypical working-class woman to be objectified or pitied. Rather we see her as she is: a quietly heroic, loving and sensitive woman whose resilience should ensure that she will persevere. It is a message well worth celebrating in a story that cries out to be widely read.

> And so she stood by the window, alone and not alone, until she heard Richard's voice calling to her from the next room. "All right," she said. "I'm coming." She took one last look, then, bracing her shoulders, went back to her children.

The Last Summer
from *Summer Lies* (2010)

Bernhard Schlink
(German writer. Born 1944)

Carol Brown Janeway
(Translator 1944–2015)

On first reading, the self-absorbed narrator of 'The Last Summer' irritated me to such a degree that I dismissed it out of hand. I was drawn back by its premise, however, and this study of a dying man's psyche slowly revealed itself to be a gem. A professor of philosophy who, unbeknownst to his family, has terminal cancer brings the extended family together at their summer house for what he intends to be a last shared holiday. He plans on taking his life at a time of his choosing, when the summer break ends and the pain of cancer becomes unendurable. The necessary cocktail of drugs has been obtained. Wife and family are oblivious to it all, excluded from his planned death just as they have perpetually been excluded from his inner life. The deception of wife and family is matched by a level of self-deception so ingrained that his efforts to finally connect and engage seem doomed from the outset. As memories surface, a lifetime of self-sabotaging behaviour is revealed. The happiness he has longed for and so desperately tried to construct has been blocked by an impenetrable self-built edifice of deceit. As he struggles with fundamental questions about life, love and happiness, the physical decay of his body accelerates under the unrelenting onslaught of cancer.

As the story begins, an invitation to return to a New York university as visiting professor is the spark that sends the central character back in time and memory. Revelatory thoughts flow as he considers his first visit to New York. These old memories reveal a life of deceit. As he considers his career, marriage, privilege and outward success, he pushes away troubling thoughts of seeking out a more fulfilling life. Any feeling that this dogged assembly of "the components of happiness" has failed to deliver is quickly suppressed. Despite this, an inkling of insight starts to break through.

> The idea of summer together, his last summer, was the idea of a last shared happiness … He had thought he'd prepared their last shared happiness. Now he wondered if once again he had only collected the components of happiness.

Self-awareness is largely absent, however. The word "shared" is like a steady refrain in Thomas Wellmer's mind but is far removed from the reality of a life lived at an emotional distance. He has chosen to be a passive observer rather than an active, open hearted participant in family life. Working hard to avoid real intimacy, he has even ensured an escape route at his summer home by renovating an old boathouse to retreat to. The deep-seated habit of withholding himself, physically and emotionally, persists despite his desire for happiness. With subtlety and skill Schlink juxtaposes the reality of the professor's life with his own delusional understanding of it. The devastating extent of the professor's self-absorption, consequent coldness, and lack of empathy for his wife and family, is gradually unmasked.

As he makes fumbling attempts to reconnect, he relishes spending time with his family. Conscious that a grandson is suffering, he longs to reach out to comfort him. The habits of a lifetime are not easily broken, however, and his efforts to find the right words fail. It is telling that he can only see his grandson's pain through the prism of his own pain. His general behaviour is so out of character that it raises eyebrows. He blocks his wife's attempt to break through the wall he has built between them. Schlink provides tantalising glimpses of the damaging impact of this lifetime of emotional deceit. Working hard to break down his wife's scepticism, he sets out to court her. The decision to lie about the motivation for his change of behaviour is a further damning betrayal. Ironically, we learn that his wife has had breast cancer and would surely respond to his diagnosis with sensitivity and real understanding. The essence of their relationship is disclosed in Schlink's spare prose.

> "You told me I'm as beautiful as I was before and you love the new breast as much as you loved the old one ... You were very understanding and very considerate, and said you didn't want to pressure me, and I should give you a signal when things were better. But when I didn't give you a signal, that was fine with you too ... Then I realised it had been the same way before the operation and nothing happened back then, either, unless I was the one to give the signal. I didn't want to give any more signals."

One of the most moving aspects of the story is the delicacy with which the progress of his cancer is laid bare. Early on, we learn how he has chosen to deal with it.

> He didn't want to be one of those sick people who know everything about their illness, who research on the Internet and in books and conversations and embarrass their doctors. Left hip, right hip – he hadn't been paying attention when the doctor told him which bones were already affected. He'd told himself he would notice soon enough.

Cancer makes its presence felt as the story progresses. As he finally overcomes his wife's scepticism and they start to make love, pain raises its ugly head.

> It had shown him that it was not only at home in his body, but that it now ruled the house. For now, it had retreated into a back room, but left the doors open in order to be right there if insufficient respect was shown.

The arrival of his closest friend brings the story's themes to a head. We learn that both men are living with different cancers and have gone on similar treatment paths, although his friend confirms he is still in remission. Their conversation is the closest the professor gets to speaking honestly about his cancer. He is careful to stop short of revealing the planned suicide. In response to his friend's query, he states:

> "It's only a matter of time before the bones give out and they crumble

and break and the pain becomes unbearable. Sometimes I get a foretaste, but things are still okay.

The ease with which his friend engages with those around him throws the professor's abject failure to connect into stark relief. His friend's relaxed charm works its magic on the professor's grandchildren as the evening progresses. In sharp contrast, the professor continues to choose to sit at a remove, observing the others interact. His thoughts light on one troubling aspect of assisted suicide.

Now he realised it wasn't simple to decide on the right evening. The longer it went on and the worse he got, the less often there would be pain-free evenings, and the more welcome and indispensable they would be. How could he relinquish such an evening to death?

The pivotal moment of the story arrives as the family reach the midway point in their holiday and the professor's sense of the fleeting nature of his last summer deepens. As he contemplates the mistakes his children are making in life, he realises that all he can do is tell them that he loves them. The pain gradually becomes so fierce that he is left with no option but to seek out his doctor for the morphine he desperately needs. On his return, he is challenged by his wife who has found the suicide cocktail and worked out its function. Her sense of betrayal, intensified by his recent deceitful attempts at intimacy, leaves little room for rapprochement. He is bewildered by his wife's sense of betrayal and unable to grasp its significance. The family leave the following morning as he struggles to understand what he has done wrong.

Self-awareness finally dawns. He sees that he has been truly happy during this last summer. He begins to listen for his family's return, convinced that it will happen. But time passes, no one comes, and he duly falls apart. Finally brought to his senses by his family's actions and with the added spur of an accident, he recognises his need for their love and support.

At first glance, this is simply a straightforward account of the dilemma one dying man finds himself in. On closer reading, it reveals itself to be a subtle and poignant meditation on universal human frailties and the harm we unwittingly inflict on ourselves and on others. It also offers an interesting perspective on the subject of assisted suicide and the human desire to die with dignity. Schlink's tale is awash with uncomfortable truths that are conveyed with the lightest of touches. His trademark spare prose is unfailingly masculine and has an innately melancholic air to it. Together with his reflective approach, it gives the story an unexpectedly powerful punch. The universality of the emotions explored compels the reader to consider lies, pretences and small betrayals, of ourselves and of others, that may be stymying our own quest to live meaningful and fulfilled lives before it is too late.

'Little Disturbances'
from *The China Factory* (2012)

Mary Costello
(*Irish writer. Born 1963*)

An Irish short story writer was always going to feature in this collection. The only difficulty I foresaw was in picking from such fertile ground. It is a rich vein in Irish literature and so many writers are masters of the genre. The tradition continues, with new short story writers constantly emerging. And yet I never expected to find the perfect Irish short story in a debut work. A first book it may be, but Costello's 'The China Factory' is the work of a writer who has quietly honed her craft over many years and emerged fully formed. Just as in Pat Barker's *Union Street*, the characteristics of great short story writing are everywhere in evidence. Echoes of Irish masters of the genre, notably John McGahern and William Trevor, can be heard. Costello's focus is on small lives that are blighted by regrets, loneliness, isolation and failure. This writer of place captures the nuances and quiet rhythms of rural life, reminding us of a rich writing heritage at every turn. Costello's writing may be built on the shoulders of Irish literary giants but she has a singular voice. Her style is minimalist – not one word is wasted. . Each sentence is precisely constructed and weighted with compressed meaning. The reader is compelled to consider every single line and to determine what has been left unsaid. Only then can meaning and truth be conceptualised. Her story of the existential threat to one man broadens out into a profound consideration of universal concerns about life and love and mortality. It is tailor-made for readers struggling with those very concerns.

We are instantly drawn into the central character's inner world, and it is a world of turmoil. Troubling thoughts and memories churning in his mind foreshadow the story's key themes. There is a sense of loss and regret in recurring, bittersweet memories of a beloved daughter, Miriam, now living in Canada. The inability to share these memories with his wife, Marie, suggests that there is something amiss in their relationship. The nagging feeling that he has failed to live fully and so has missed out on life's hidden possibilities stretches right back in time to his daughter's early childhood. The spark that has ignited this hotbed of anxieties is revealed during a breakfast conversation between husband and wife. Costello's dialogue rings with authenticity. So much is revealed in glances and in what is left unsaid. We learn that medical test results await at the doctor's surgery, results that he has no desire to hear. Intuitively he already knows what it will mean for him but, determined to postpone facing the inevitable, works to persuade his wife to go in his stead. The word *cancer* is never mentioned. Instead, not unexpectedly for a man of his generation and community, we are told:

> The sickness had been inside him for months.

Awareness of approaching death has prompted him to reassess his life. Bewilderment and sadness threaten to overwhelm him as he considers how a marriage that started out with such promise has changed over time, with real connection dissipating and love fading. He remembers the passionate love that first brought them together. Costello's beautifully constructed sentences suggest that hope, however faint, still exists for their marriage. Marie's inner life is never presented, but her words and actions suggest a level of awareness of her husband's anxieties and a desire to help. Costello gently nudges the reader to wonder what caused the apparent estrangement of father and daughter. When Marie raises the subject of Miriam, who is in the father's thoughts at that very moment, it prompts a sharing of old parental worries for a delicate and sensitive child. This conversation concludes with Marie's telling line:

> "I don't know where she got it ... all that fainting, all that feeling."

We can only infer from Costello's rather touching words that father and daughter share this trait of struggling with emotions that they find difficult to express and almost impossible to manage. As he continues to brood about his marital relationship and the missteps taken over a lifetime, Marie departs to keep the doctor's appointment. In her absence he considers how the looming threat to his life has heightened his consciousness of the physical world.

The acute sense of his own mortality has unleashed a veritable tsunami of memories, thoughts and feelings that manifest in vivid dreams in which death is a steady refrain. The slaughter of farm animals, a routine part of the cycle of his farming life, is a recurring motif. One dream suggests that the lamb at his mercy, the lamb who has been metaphorically slaughtered, is his daughter Miriam. When the detail of his parental betrayal is exposed, it would seem to merit the weight of guilt and regret that he carries. His fateful actions broke his daughter's heart and, consequently, tore the family apart. For a man of his time and place, the motivation is utterly believable. Costello fleshes out the character so well that the reader understands and empathises with this flawed human being. The consequence of his abject parental failure is immense suffering. Miriam is the long-lost lamb that he grieves for, a grief that the presence of his other adult children cannot alleviate.

As his wife's return from the doctor nears and the story moves to a conclusion, Costello creates a realistic and powerful picture of what it is like to endure dread and fear in isolation. Symbolism is used to great effect, with glimmers of hope delicately woven into the pervading sense of doom as he waits for a cancer prognosis that intuitively he knows will deliver the very worst news.

> A white butterfly lands on a flower. He had never noticed butterflies or flowers much before … A cloud gathers directly above him, and seems to hang there for a minute. It starts to mushroom out then. He has the feeling that it will lower itself down over him. His heart thumps faster. He feels some danger close by, as if the cloud has come to pester him or question him, and when he has no answers, it will press down on him and enclose him and smother him. He closes his eyes tight and then, for no reason, he turns his head and there among Marie's red dahlias is the white butterfly. He watches its wings moving. He feels a little release, as if the cloud is lifting. He feels some goodness, and that it is coming from the butterfly. He watches it flitting among the flowers. For a second he is free. Then his breath catches and he thinks how something of Marie always revives him. He feels himself break.

The white butterfly is an important symbol in many cultures. In Irish folklore it represents the soul of the dead waiting to cross to the next world and is seen as a bearer of good luck. That the butterfly is set among Marie's flowers is a poignant reminder of how deeply he yearns to reconnect with his wife and bridge the chasm that has developed between them. His yearning to be safe and secure manifests in recurring references to a deep fear of the pull of water. When the moment finally arrives and the feared medical news passes from wife to husband, it is an object lesson in great storytelling.

The nature of the "little disturbances" that are haunting this lonely and emotionally isolated man are brought to light by the story's end. Although there may be hardly a ripple visible on the surface, his inner self is a maelstrom of feelings, reminding the reader of the intended irony in the story's title. He is suffused with fear and dread. A feeling that death is approaching has compelled him to consider the life he has lived and thereby has unleashed intense feelings of regret, guilt and loss. The sense of having failed to fully embrace life and love unconditionally has left him yearning to address his deepest concerns and find some semblance of peace. On his wife's return, his worst fears are confirmed but, in an inspired move, Costello chooses to conclude with signs of resignation, acceptance and even hope. It is the hope that comes from the examined life and the acuity it bestows.

> He will no longer be afraid to say things. When night comes they will lie down and he will tell her that she has never changed and that her blue-grey eyes remind him of a wolf's. He will tell her that there was always some want in him and he is afraid of almost everything right now. He will ask her to send for Miriam. He will remind her that the front of the graveyard gets waterlogged in winter, and to go well back towards the end. *Pick a dry grave for me*, he will say. *Don't bury me in water.*

Costello's 'Little Disturbances' deals with the enormity of the emotional aspects of the cancer experience with such subtlety and skill that it was a natural choice for this collection. The reader can relate to the intensity and complexity of one man's inner life as he grapples with his fate. I was struck by many interesting similarities to themes explored by Alice Munro and Leo Tolstoy. Costello's place in *The Breath of Consolation* was absolutely guaranteed by that lovely glimmer of hope in the story's closing lines. There is a recognition of the universal desire for a meaningful and fulfilled life, however small and insignificant that life may outwardly appear to be, and a reminder that even in the face of death, the human capacity to search for self-understanding, and to respond to the examined life accordingly, is incredibly powerful. For those living and dying with cancer *Little Disturbances* is a welcome reminder that we are not alone in our struggle for self-understanding and acceptance. Somehow, this one story securely anchors the reader's determination to persevere, even if death is approaching. Costello prompts us to keep in mind that it is never too late to recover hope and be at peace with fate.

The Death of Ivan Ilyich (1886)

Leo Tolstoy
(Russian writer 1828–1910)

Peter Carson
(English Translator 1938–2013)

At the very moment that this book was conceived, *The Death of Ivan Ilyich* was the only fictional work that I knew with absolute certainty had to feature. Tolstoy's masterful novella has no equal for those enduring the grim realities of cancer and grappling with making sense not only of suffering and death, but also of life. His existential reflections on the meaning of life in the context of the inevitability of death remain as fresh, pertinent and clear as the day they were written. Tolstoy initially shows us death through the eyes of the living and then moves the perspective to death as it is experienced by one flawed, dying man. He compels the reader to take a difficult and intimate journey into Ivan's personal nightmare. It is a deeply moving depiction of the horrors of the dying process and the mounting physical and psychological pain endured. The clue to the terrors experienced by Ivan in facing his mortality lies in the way he chose to live and so Tolstoy brings us on a journey through that life.

Ivan Ilyich's world of work, family, colleagues and his wider social circle is laid bare. Tolstoy's description of that world rings as true for modern readers as it did for his contemporaries. Human nature hasn't changed and so Ivan Ilyich is instantly recognisable. He is an everyman character, small-minded and never satisfied with what he has. In telling Ivan's universal story, Tolstoy takes a cold, hard look not only at death but at human nature. Ivan Ilyich's death is recounted at the start of the novel in all its excruciating detail but Tolstoy also reveals his character's self-interested, materialistic and shallow world. His death is nothing more to his colleagues than an immediate inconvenience, quickly followed by an opportunity for career progress. The routine expressions of grief ring hollow.

> Ivan Ilyich was a colleague of the gentlemen meeting there and they all liked him ... on hearing of Ivan Ilyich's death, the first thought of each of the gentlemen meeting in the room was of the significance the death might have for the transfer or promotion of the members themselves or their friends.

When Ivan's wife takes his closest friend aside as he leaves the room where Ivan has been laid out, it is not to mourn her husband. Rather, it is to talk about what she herself has gone through and to inquire about her pension.

> "Did he suffer very much?" Pyotr Ivanovich asked. "Oh. Terribly! At the end he never stopped screaming, not for minutes, for hours. For three whole days he screamed without drawing breath. It was unbearable. I can't understand how I bore it; one could hear it from three doors away. Oh, what I've been through!"

A quite well-regarded, middle-aged judge, Ivan's focus has always been fixed on climbing the career and the social ladder. With shallow relationships and an empty and fractious marriage, Ivan has lived a selfish, materialistic and narrow life, devoid of introspection.

A seemingly minor injury develops into a serious matter for which doctors have conflicting diagnoses and useless prescriptions. Known for strongly disliking the medical profession, Tolstoy portrays Ivan's doctors as uncaring and devoid of empathy and compassion. They also fail to do anything meaningful to help him. Tolstoy draws a parallel between their attitude and the dismissive way Ivan himself has treated those brought before him in court. A clear diagnosis is never given for Ivan's illness. This has long been the subject of discussion among scholars who now mostly agree that Tolstoy's description indicates cancer. There is no doubt that Tolstoy is purposely vague as he is making the point that the actual diagnosis is irrelevant. It does not change the fact that Ivan is dying and is only a distraction from what the focus should be on, i.e. the dying process. When medicine fails, Ivan turns in despair to homeopathy and then to religious relics but finds them equally useless. How little has changed! Ivan soon realises that he is dying.

> There was light and now there's darkness. I was here and now I'm going there! Where? A chill came over him, his breathing stopped. He could only hear the beating of his heart.

He also recognises that most of his family and friends refuse to acknowledge his reality and engage in deceitful behaviour, regarding the dying process as an inconvenience. Ivan's world shrinks to his study as his body degenerates. He experiences increasing pain, physical indignities, isolation, terror and deep unhappiness.

> Whether it was morning or evening, Friday or Sunday, was immaterial, it was all one and the same: the gnawing, agonising pain that didn't abate for a moment; the consciousness of life departing without hope but still not yet departed; the same terrible, hateful death advancing, which was the only reality, and always the same lie.

His only relief and consolation come from the company of Gerasim, a young peasant servant who does not deny reality but instead openly acknowledges that Ivan is dying. Gerasim offers real compassion and deals with the physical unpleasantness involved in caring for Ivan. It is not Ivan's doctors but this servant who discovers a practical way to physically ease Ivan's pain, at no little physical cost to himself. In this way, the reader is shown how an authentic life is lived. Gerasim offers truth, empathy, compassion and practical comfort to the dying man. It is not accidental that Ivan begins to question his own life when Gerasim is present.

> ... but even more terrible than his physical sufferings were his mental sufferings, and there was his chief torment ... as he looked at Gerasim's sleepy, good-natured face with its high cheekbones, there suddenly had entered his head the thought: *But what if in actual fact all my life, my conscious life, has been 'wrong?'*

As he considers how he has lived, he moves from at first believing that he has lived rightly to gradually acknowledging that he has deluded himself and has in fact lived an artificial life, far removed from meaningful and truthful relationships. An inner life has simply not existed. He has also lived without generosity, kindness or empathy. Instead, his focus has been on his own needs, petty vanities and empty social and career ambitions.

Ivan's moment of epiphany comes as he realises that he has lived an empty life but that it is still open to him to choose to live authentically even if it is only in his last moments. Although he has fought against looking down into the abyss, the reality of the dying process and the psychological journey he has taken finally enable him to overcome his fears. He faces death with equanimity. It is no surprise that this moment comes when he feels his grief-stricken son kissing his hand and sees his wife weeping. Ivan is moved, feels compassion for his family and understands that his death will be a release for them. He tries to ask for forgiveness. The story ends with a wonderfully human, vivid and truthful portrait of physical death. No doubt it reflects Tolstoy's long personal experience of loss, including the deaths of many children. Tolstoy mirrors words Ivan used when he first recognised that he was dying.

> Where was death? What death? There was no fear, because there was no death.
> Instead of death there was light.
> "So that's it!" he suddenly said aloud. "Such joy!"
> For him all this took place in a moment, and the significance of this moment didn't change. For those there his death agony lasted two hours more. Something bubbled in his chest; his emaciated body shivered. Then the gurgling and wheezing became less and less frequent.
> "It is finished!" Someone said above him.
> He heard these words and repeated them in his heart.
> "Death is finished," he said to himself. "It is no more."
> He breathed in, stopped halfway, stretched himself, and died.

Tolstoy demonstrates his mastery of the written word as he moves readers from a judgemental and critical view of Ivan to a compassionate understanding of his struggles and a recognition that we ourselves are not so different. Tolstoy reminds us that we are subject to the same forces, vulnerable to the same delusions, and just as capable of living a meaningless life. He nudges us to consider our own behaviour and to reflect on who we are and how we are choosing to use our limited time in this world. Tolstoy was obsessed with death and with issues of morality. The reader can clearly see his moralist viewpoint in his writing. His challenge to readers is really the only one worth taking on: he tells us not to fear death but to recognise its inevitability and to consider instead what constitutes an authentic life. He entreats us to choose to live our lives fully and truthfully.

The rationale for placing Tolstoy's work last in this section was three-fold. Firstly, I wanted to bookend my recommendations with my two absolute favourites. Secondly, I feared that placing a 19th-Century writer first might be off-putting for some readers. As a librarian I know only too well that classic writers are not as widely read as they deserve to be, or indeed as readers claim. Lastly and most importantly, Tolstoy's novella is a reminder that rich literature offers something fresh, thought-provoking and satisfying – regardless of its form, origin, or the age in which it's read. Tolstoy hones in with a forensic eye on the universal questions that trouble every human being dealing with serious illness. He nudges us to think about what really matters, and who we choose to be. Ultimately, *The Death of Ivan Ilych* consoles us, with its inspiring message that hope can be recovered and serenity achieved. After all, if a small-minded and self-absorbed man like Ivan Ilych can yearn for and finally achieve serenity, surely that possibility exists within all of us.

PART 5

Fabulous Endings

Introduction

James Baldwin, a singular writer lost too soon to us because of cancer, described the transformative power of literature.

> You write in order to change the world, knowing perfectly well that you probably can't, but also knowing that literature is indispensable to the world … The world changes according to the way people see it, and if you alter, even by a millimeter, the way … people look at reality, then you can change it.

Outside of the four key genres, just six outstanding books demanded inclusion in this gathering of great cancer literature. All are ground-breaking classics written by natural storytellers and have the capacity to transform how we respond to cancer.

The first two books are critically acclaimed explorations of the socio-political, economic and cultural landscape that shaped the history of cancer science and medicine. Many authors have attempted to tackle this subject. None have come close to the epic scope, masterful research, and remarkable writing of Siddhartha Mukherjee and Clifton Leaf. The possibility of eradicating cancer forever is the fundamental issue that haunts both writers. For two books that cover similar territory, the contrast in their approaches and conclusions is striking. Yet we shouldn't be surprised by this, given their very different backgrounds. Mukherjee is a cancer physician and researcher. Leaf is an investigative journalist and cancer survivor. Both writers deliver real insights into the history of cancer but also clear-eyed assessments of what the future may hold. Moreover, how thrilling to find that homage is paid to the outstanding contributions of two people with strong Irish connections. Leaf honours the ground-breaking research of the "one-eyed Irish surgeon" Denis

Burkitt. Mukherjee recognises the pioneering work of Mary Lasker, a woman who publicly acknowledged the formative influence of her Irish mother. Both books emancipate the reader by enhancing our understanding of this terrible disease.

The profound injustices that exist in the medical science and cancer care worlds, with catastrophic consequences for the marginalised, are exposed in Rebecca Skloot's compelling narrative. The story of Henrietta Lacks and her transformative immortal cell line is truly extraordinary. No one who reads this book could doubt that equity and human rights must be placed at the heart of global healthcare and scientific research.

On my odyssey through cancer literature, I stumbled upon an academic scholar and cancer survivor who shares my conviction that cancer literature has the power to heal. Susan Gubar's valuable work is a useful manual for those who want to write about their personal cancer experience. It is also a fascinating guide to reading cancer literature. Although quite different in tone, content and structure, it is hugely complementary to this work.

There was never any doubt that C.S. Lewis's classic of grief literature would feature in this last section. A powerful interrogation of love, loss, suffering, and religious faith, *A Grief Observed* is full of heart and wisdom. Readers in crisis because of cancer will find great solace in Lewis's meditative work.

There is something quite magical in how my journey through cancer literature brought me full circle. The earliest root of my odyssey through great books about the disease lies in a fruitless search for words that would give solace to the dying Irish writer Nuala O'Faolain. It ended with the discovery of the perfect work, albeit one published seven years after her death. Oliver Sacks's *Gratitude* never fails to console me when darkness and dread threaten. For those who are devoid of hope and feel life is drained of meaning, Sacks's "statement of departure" has the power to heal and console.

The Emperor of All Maladies: A Biography of Cancer (2010)

Siddhartha Mukherjee

(Indian American writer. Born 1970)

Living with an incurable blood cancer has made every personal milestone since treatment a cause for mindful celebration. In May 2018, by sheer good luck, I marked my second birthday in remission by attending a lecture in Dublin given by an author whom I hugely admire but never imagined I'd hear speak in person. Siddhartha Mukherjee is a blood cancer physician, researcher, and gifted writer. His Pulitzer Prize-winning book *The Emperor of All Maladies* made an extraordinary impact on me when I first read it, shortly after my cancer diagnosis in 2014. I am always a little wary of books that receive uniformly rave reviews but Mukherjee's work lives up to all the hype. It is epic, both in ambition and in execution. His stated aim at the outset is to answer two formidable and interlinked questions:

> Is cancer's end conceivable in the future? Is it possible to eradicate this disease from our bodies and societies forever?

I was instantly hooked by his audacious ambition, eager to discover how he would explore cancer's history, where it would lead, and what conclusions would result.

In Mukherjee's heroic quest for an answer, we are brought on a meticulously researched journey through the history of cancer science and medicine and the socio-political, economic and cultural landscape that shaped it. It is a roller coaster of a ride, from the earliest descriptions of cancer in an ancient Egyptian manuscript through to the development of the dominant treatment regimens of surgery, radiation and chemotherapy, and finally on to the era of targeted molecular therapy. The passion, drive and ambition of two key figures lie at the very heart of the story – the scientist Sidney Farber and the political lobbyist and philanthropist Mary Lasker. Unleashing a crusade for a national response to cancer, their gargantuan joint effort eventually resulted in the declaration of a War on Cancer in the U.S. in 1971. It was a transformative moment, not least for how it forever embedded the language of war into the way we think and communicate about cancer. What began with such promise soon descended into what Mukherjee describes as a War *Within* Cancer. And yet, even during this fraught period, advances continued to be made. The integration of preventive measures and multiple treatment types, with hormonal therapy now added to the arsenal, delivered qualified successes. Bolstered by second-wave feminism in the 1970s and the response to the AIDS epidemic in the 1980s, the era of effective patient advocacy finally dawned. With the emergence of the palliative care movement, appropriate end-of-life care for the terminally ill became a reality. The final seismic shift examined is the discovery that cancer is the result of a process of genetic mutations that can be targeted with largely non-toxic molecular therapy.

On the face of it, and for the layperson at least, this is a book that should not work. It is a dense read, weighed down with scientific information. It is daunting at first, both in scale and in complexity. For those of us struggling with cancer, there are moments that hit such a raw nerve that it is sometimes difficult to keep going. The appalling history of paternalistic and misogynistic behaviour in cancer medicine is deeply unsettling. (Perhaps Irish women are particularly sensitive to accounts of medical misogyny having endured a long litany of such cases, culminating in the ongoing Cervical Check cancer scandal.) Finally, leukaemia is placed centre stage. For the reader living with blood cancer this is challenging if not unexpected. Not only is leukaemia the focus of Mukherjee's career but it has played, and continues to play, a crucial role in cancer research.

Despite such misgivings, Mukherjee's book held this reader's attention. Indeed, by the end of the story, I was enthralled. The reason is simple. Mukherjee writes remarkably well. The key facets of great writing are all present. The narrative is skilfully and coherently structured and well-paced.

Mukherjee's ability to juggle so many roles is truly remarkable. He is, by turns, the attentive doctor describing the experiences of patients under his care; the historian enraptured by his subject; the scientist capable of producing clear explanations of complex concepts; the eager biographer bringing characters memorably to life; the teacher who refuses to "dumb down" his subject yet still succeeds in holding and stimulating his audience; the human being disturbed by the cancer conundrum and our shared fragility in the face of its destructive power. Above all, Mukherjee is the writer and storyteller who revels in words and whose writing reflects a deep knowledge and love of literature. Literary allusions abound, adding depth and meaning, and literary quotations feature prominently. But it is Mukherjee's unmistakable writing style that captivates. The joy of reading *The Emperor of All Maladies* rests on the successful fusion of all of these elements.

The soul of Mukherjee's work lies in a large cast of real-life characters, brought vividly to life through the alchemy of his words. The reader encounters patients, advocates, activists and a pioneering group of scientists, doctors and medical students. Wisely, Mukherjee places the patient centre stage. He signposts this intention from the get-go with a poignant dedication to Robert Sandler, a toddler treated by Sidney Farber in 1948 who, after a brief remission, died of leukaemia. The narrative thread of Carla Reed's evolving cancer journey under Mukherjee's care is introduced at the very start. As the book progresses, we follow her from diagnosis through treatment for acute leukaemia and onto a prolonged remission. Key figures from the early days of patient advocacy – Rachel Carson, Rose Kushner and Betty Rollin – appear only briefly but shine brightly. Other patient cases featured are carefully chosen to represent a spectrum of survivors whose cancer was controlled or cured by a range of treatments. The often-horrific impact and long term effects of treatment are not ignored, as a meeting Mukherjee had with a woman cured of childhood leukaemia illustrates.

> I sensed a shiver running through her body, as if even today, forty-five years after her ordeal, the memory haunts her viscerally.

The tone throughout is compassionate and empathetic but also somewhat emotionally disconnected. This is not at all surprising given that it seems to be a survival mechanism common among haematologists and oncologists. The care Mukherjee has poured into this work is evident throughout, not least in how he brings his book to a close with a patient's story that is an appropriate symbol of the current state of the cancer experience. He recounts Germaine Berne's tortuous six-year struggle with cancer and the self-advocacy role that she adopted in the search for a reprieve. How her personal life was transformed by cancer is touched on, before that fateful moment arrives when there is nowhere left to turn and it is finally time to accept approaching death. Although I am deeply uncomfortable with the language of cancer heroism, there is no mistaking Mukherjee's sincere regard for patients. Indeed, at his Dublin lecture and for an audience largely made up of doctors and medical students, he reiterated that view which is captured so beautifully in the following extract.

> But the story of leukaemia – the story of cancer – isn't the story of doctors who struggle and survive, moving from one institution to another. It is the story of patients who struggle and survive, moving from one embankment of illness to another. Resilience, inventiveness, and survivorship – qualities often ascribed to great physicians – are reflected qualities, emanating first from those who struggle with illness and only then mirrored by those who treat them.

Despite the profusion of doctors and scientists that feature in the book, Mukherjee manages to set each and every one apart. His observational and descriptive powers ensure that many are seared forever into this reader's memory. The father of chemotherapy, Sidney Farber, is:

> ... formal, precise, and meticulous, starched in his appearance and his mannerisms and commanding in presence ... nicknamed Four-Button Sid for his propensity for wearing formal suits to his classes.

John Hunter, an 18th-century Scottish surgeon and a key figure in the development of surgery as a cancer treatment, is the "immaculate anatomist". A pioneer in radiation oncology, Émil Grubbé, is "flamboyant, adventurous, and fiercely inventive". We are told that Thomas Hodgkin, discoverer of Hodgkin lymphoma, looks like a character from an Edward Lear poem. The depiction of the "two Emils" – Freireich and Frei – who in the early 1960s created a successful chemotherapy programme for leukaemia, is touchingly human.

Freireich was flamboyant, hot-tempered, and adventurous. He spoke

> quickly, often explosively, with a booming voice ... If Freireich had been a character in a film, he would have needed a cinematic foil, a Laurel to his Hardy or a Felix to his Oscar ...Where Freireich was brusque and flamboyant, impulsive to a fault, and passionate about every detail, Frei was cool, composed, and cautious, a poised negotiator who preferred to work backstage ... He was charming, soft-spoken, and careful ...

There is one character that this reader would like to forget but unfortunately never will. William Halsted was an American surgeon whose radical mastectomies permanently disfigured women's bodies. Hugely influential, he shaped a generation of surgeons in his image and in so doing effectively silenced for years dissenting voices who argued for a far less radical approach. Who could resist Mukherjee's perceptive depiction of this high- functioning but drug-addicted surgeon?

> Childless, socially awkward, formal, and notoriously reclusive ... He was fascinated by anatomy. This fascination, like many of Halsted's other interests in his later years – purebred dogs, horses, starched tablecloths, linen shirts, Parisian leather shoes, and immaculate sutures – soon grew into an obsessive quest ...

Mukherjee celebrates the achievements of the many "outsiders", doctors and scientists (Sidney Farber included), who were not part of an elite inner circle yet still made seismic advances in the history of cancer medicine and research. Outstanding women include Lucy Wills, whose discovery of the link between vitamins, bone marrow and normal blood impacted on Farber's efforts to treat childhood leukaemia. The visionary Cicely Saunders, an English nurse whose childhood experiences made her especially sensitive to the feelings of outsiders, became a doctor specifically to help dying patients, and went on to establish the palliative care movement that transformed the world of the terminally ill. The first oncologist to use chemotherapy to cure cancer in adults was a Chinese American, Min Chiu Li, who in 1957 lost his job for his efforts but was ultimately vindicated. George Papanicolaou, a Greek scientist who developed the "Pap smear" test and in so doing revolutionised the early detection of cervical cancer, was initially refused American medical registration and forced to work in a succession of low paid, menial jobs on his arrival in New York. In a world where the spectre of xenophobic and nationalistic politics looms large and where difference is all too often feared, Mukherjee's message is subtle but important. The role that individuals of different ethnicities, genders, religions, cultures, racial and social backgrounds have played in the development of cancer treatment has been, and continues to be, immense.

Many of the remarkable people who populate *The Emperor of All Maladies* could legitimately claim the title of hero. If such a title could be awarded to just one person, then it should by rights go to the extraordinary Mary Lasker. She is of course one of the two key figures that lie at the very heart of Mukherjee's work. He describes the coming together of Sidney Farber and Mary Lasker as "like the meeting of two stranded travellers, each carrying one half of a map". It is noteworthy that in some reviews of Mukherjee's work, Mary Lasker's name is either not mentioned at all or simply noted in passing, with all the emphasis being placed on Farber and other doctors and scientists. Such reviews effectively demote her. The depth and breadth of her achievements in the decades-long efforts to transform the world of cancer politically and scientifically deserve, indeed demand, proper recognition. Happily, Mukherjee gives it, paying homage magnificently.

> Farber needed a colossal force behind him ... Real money, and the real power to transform, still lay under congressional control ... There was, he knew, one person who possessed the energy, resources, and passion for the project: a pugnacious New Yorker who had declared it her personal mission to transform the geography of American health through group-building, lobbying, and political action ... Wealthy, politically savvy, well connected, she lunched with the Rockefellers, danced with the Trumans, dined with the Kennedys, and called Lady Bird Johnson by her first name ... This idea – of transforming the landscape of American medical research using political lobbying and fund-raising at an unprecedented scale – electrified her.

Mukherjee touches on Lasker's Irish roots. From the Mary Lasker Papers held in Columbia University it is clear that her Irish mother, Sara Johnson Woodard, was the formative influence on Lasker's life. In a multitude of ways, Lasker followed a path that was forged for her by her enterprising mother. An Ulster Methodist, Sara Johnson emigrated to Canada in the 1880s, on her own and without qualifications, aged just seventeen. She then moved to the

U.S., and through a career in sales, became the highest paid woman in Chicago. Following her marriage she settled in Watertown, Wisconsin. Her extensive list of accomplishments includes the establishment of Watertown public library, a feat achieved in co-operation with the Carnegie Foundation. The phrase "like mother, like daughter" certainly applies to Sara and Mary. Perhaps the most endearing explanation of how influential Mary Lasker was can be found in Senator Ted Kennedy's Congressional speech on the occasion of her death in 1994.

> "When I first came to the Senate, I remember very clearly the advice that President Kennedy gave me. 'Have lunch with medical school professors, have dinner with Nobel Prize winners, but if you really want to know about what needs to be done in medical research in America, have a talk with Mary Lasker.'" (Congressional Record Feb 23rd, 1994)

Mukherjee's meditative and exhaustive survey of the history of cancer ends with a predictably nuanced, realistic, but also cautiously optimistic response to the questions posed at the outset. He suggests that there is a need to redefine what victory over cancer should look like. Given cancer's heterogeneity and how entrenched it is in our very being, more modest goals are needed. He suggests that cancer has no universal "off" switch to be discovered. Instead, the focus should be placed on putting cancer on hold; slowing or stopping its growth; and developing innovative treatments to support patients in outliving their cancer. In effect, he suggests that we should be working to prolong life rather than striving to eliminate death.

> Perhaps cancer, the scrappy, fecund, invasive, adaptable twin to our own scrappy, fecund, invasive, adaptable cells and genes, is impossible to disconnect from our bodies …With cancer, where no simple, universal, or definitive cure is in sight – and is never likely to be – the past is constantly conversing with the future. Old observations crystallise into new theories; time past is always contained in time future … But much about this battle will remain the same: the relentlessness, the inventiveness, the resilience, the queasy pivoting between defeatism and hope, the hypnotic drive for universal solutions, the disappointment of defeat, the arrogance and the hubris.

The Emperor of All Maladies is an erudite chronicle but also a riveting read, brimming with fascinating characters. Mukherjee takes us on a labyrinthine journey that absorbs our full attention from beginning to end. We are left with a far better understanding of cancer, and of the incredible complexity of treating such a heterogeneous disease. Mukherjee offers a glimpse of the future, with the cat-and-mouse game continuing and scientists and doctors, like Lewis Carroll's Red Queen, running just to stay in the same place. It is a sobering and somewhat unsettling conclusion to a remarkable book. My copy, personally signed by Siddhartha Mukherjee in the Royal College of Surgeons in Dublin, and on my birthday no less, will forever be cherished.

The Truth in Small Doses: Why We're Losing the War on Cancer – and How to Win It (2013)

Clifton Leaf

(American writer. Born 1963)

Over the last decade, and indeed since the publication of Siddhartha Mukherjee's *The Emperor of All Maladies*, the conversation around cancer has been shaped by just a handful of critically acclaimed books by medical professors, science writers and journalists. Tough questions are posed around four central issues: the terrifying human cost of cancer; the state of cancer research; the likelihood of success in eradicating this heterogeneous disease; and what, if anything, needs to change if that goal is to be met swiftly and decisively. Leaf's masterful book *The Truth in Small Doses* transcends all others in addressing these questions. He dares to plot a way forward that, if taken, might just succeed in transforming cancer care and move it off a well-worn path that is failing spectacularly to lead to the desired results.

Leaf is an investigative journalist who spent the best part of a decade researching the world of cancer. Although his focus is on America, Leaf's findings have global ramifications as America's cancer culture is so dominant, with many countries across the world following its lead. With an outsider's eye, he brings clarity to the complex and murky mix of science, medicine, history, politics, pharma and other sectoral interests that make up the cancer story. The critical fault lines that are undermining the global effort to eradicate cancer are unearthed and then powerfully critiqued. Leaf's voice is multi-layered and compelling. We hear the voice of the thorough, skilful and determined journalist who is also a natural storyteller. We also listen to the cancer survivor, outraged by how the current system is failing patients and frustrated by the lack of honesty about the true state of play. Finally, there is an advocate's urgency in his clear, eloquent call for action.

The scientific revolution of targeted drug therapies was the spark that lit Leaf's interest in cancer reporting. From the mid-1990s onward, drugs such as Avastin, Herceptin and Gleevec seemed to herald an end to the cancer war. Leaf therefore anticipated reporting on a story of brilliant advances, surefootedly moving towards ultimate success. As one would expect from a financial journalist, his research started with a close examination of the numbers. What the scientific data revealed, however, was a stark and ever-worsening reality.

> There was a profound disconnect between the rhetoric of top management and the numbers. NCI officials and leading oncologists were talking about 'steady progress' and 'turned corners' and 'breakthroughs', but the statistics told a far more depressing tale ... For the past several decades, reports of shining advances in cancer biology and treatment have streamed into newspapers, magazines, and television sets the world over. But during that time, there has been only minor change in the prospects for most people with active disease: survival numbers have barely improved; new cases keep mounting; death counts continue to rise ... it takes no leap of logic to conclude that our strategy is flawed. All it takes is a little counting.

The dawning realisation that the war on cancer is in serious trouble, and that this is down to a dysfunctional cancer culture, inspired Leaf to undertake a nine-year quest with one key question at its heart: How did we get here? In his view, answering that question was the route to understanding the challenge ahead. Only then could major issues be tackled and the system realigned to make cancer's eradication truly feasible.

Leaf begins his book with an exhaustive assessment of the growing cancer burden. He reveals how the use of scientific data is misleading and obscures the big picture. The denial of what the scientific data actually tells us is so ingrained in cancer culture that even well-respected statisticians who openly challenge incorrect assumptions about progress risk being side-lined. This cavalier attitude to truth is deeply rooted. Leaf's concern about the damaging cultural disconnect from honesty in the cancer world influenced his choice of book title. It is taken from a pamphlet published in 1959 advising doctors that their best approach is to trickle out information to cancer patients, offering "the truth in small doses". Ireland's recent cervical cancer scandal would only seem to confirm that the culture of withholding the truth from cancer patients persists and is deeply embedded well beyond American shores.

Whilst acknowledging the many achievements that have occurred over past decades, including the phenomenal successes with childhood cancers, Leaf questions the assumption that the route to victory over cancer lies in finding cures. He argues that far more effort needs to be directed at cancer prevention, reminding us that treatment is the greatest cancer burden of all. The immense costs paid by patients, carers and families go way beyond cancer's financial millstone. Yet these costs are largely hidden and unaccounted for in statistics.

> Cancer treatment can feel like an exhausting board game come to life, a route in which every other square requires a new blood test, scan, or X-Ray, where the path is stalled by interminable waiting room waits, insurance forms, and unanswered questions. For many patients, there is little difference between treatment and disease. Pain from one melds into pain from the other; fear of the cancer is subsumed, at times, by the immediate dread of a brutal drug or procedure. They are the two faces of the same ordeal … Nor, for many people, does the emotional trauma end with the final round of treatment. The diagnosis continues to tow behind it the nag of uncertainty, whispering anew with each swollen gland, fever, or malaise. Even when the cancer is truly gone, even when the scans are clean, it can seem that the 'cure' is held in an escrow of medical testing and follow-up.

Leaf gives a human face to the treatment burden by offering a brief but poignant glimpse into his family's experience. As he outlines his mother's long struggle with a rare cancer and his own treatment for Hodgkin lymphoma as a teenager, he chooses to shine the spotlight on his father's suffering and the devastating and far-reaching ramifications of treatment.

The statistics demonstrate that soaring numbers are being diagnosed and deaths are continuing at a frightening pace despite eye-watering levels of expenditure on cancer research and treatment. Leaf convincingly argues that the focus needs to go on anticipating, finding and destroying cancer in its earliest developmental stages. This challenging task demands wise investment in research on pre-emptive measures including carcinogenesis, screening and prevention. In reality, the research balance is dangerously skewed, with resources continuing to pour into new drug development for late-stage disease. Leaf's view is that nothing less than a paradigm shift will ensure that anticipating, finding and destroying *first* cancer cells is pursued at least as aggressively as chasing cancer in progressive and late-stage disease.

Unlike with recent global financial catastrophes, Leaf finds no villains in the international cancer story. Rather, he concludes that the core of the problem is systemic. As his comprehensive notes and references demonstrate, his overall assessment has in fact already been arrived at by many cancer world leaders. Yet little has been done to resolve the problem and nothing of substance has changed over decades. Leaf traces cancer culture's dysfunctional nature back to the 1971 legislation that launched the war on cancer. The Act bore little relation to the original measure pioneered by Farber and Lasker and introduced by Ted Kennedy. In fact, the 1971 Act spawned a massive cancer industry that benefits from monumental financial investment but is risk-averse, bureaucratic, and ultra-conservative.

> The war on cancer was not a war at all ... there were no deadlines, no accountability, no risk, no leaps into the unknown, no dark side of the moon ... no great crusade ... There was simply more money to spend.

The cancer industry was plagued from the outset by an absence of vision, leadership and effective management. Over decades, the system has evolved into one that wastes invaluable scientists' time in laborious grant application processes and resultant paperwork. Critically, little if any incentive is offered for national or international collaboration. Year after year, funding is overwhelmingly directed to established institutions and low-risk research, whilst young researchers struggle to attract resources. Any researcher who wants to focus on provocative or novel areas finds funding virtually impossible to source. Innovation is stifled and research that is narrowly focused on incremental improvements is encouraged. In consequence, cancer drug development produces many 'me-too' drugs with limited value for patients and with prices that are pushed up to unaffordable levels. Clinical trials have modest ambitions and paralysing regulations and are slow to get up and running. The vast majority continue to fail. Those that do succeed frequently extend life only by a few months and at huge cost. In short, it is a system in crisis. Leaf makes a powerful case for the dismantling of existing micromanagement and mismanagement systems of cancer research, arguing that what is desperately needed are quantum leaps not tiny steps forward.

In searching for an archetype for how cancer research *should* work, Leaf turns to the incredible story of a "one-eyed Irish surgeon" who was born near Enniskillen in 1911 and educated at Trinity College Dublin. Denis Burkitt made a unique and remarkable contribution to cancer research. He discovered a lethal and fast-growing paediatric lymphoma and mapped its geographic distribution through a formidable 'tumour safari' across the continent of Africa with two colleagues in the early 1960s. Laughably miniscule funding did not deter him. He established a genuine and truly international collaborative effort over many years, enlisting the help of doctors and scientists across disciplines and countries who freely shared tumour samples, data and information. All this took place long before the computer age or indeed the start of the war on cancer. Burkitt was prepared to act when he saw young lives at stake and took educated risks to treat his patients, saving lives in the process. Ever modest, Burkitt described his role as that of "a launching pad from which others can fire their rockets".

> Burkitt taught the world how powerful true scientific collaboration can be. Far-flung investigators, working together, unravelled a cancer mystery that no single scientist would ever have solved on his own. It's a lesson that remains as essential today as ever.

Leaf suggests that the adoption of a Burkitt model of cancer research would encourage novel thinking, free up the sharing of ideas and data, and enable pioneering researchers to take educated, risky but absolutely necessary leaps of faith.

Uniquely, Leaf also recognises and writes about the largely untapped potential of patient advocacy. Establishing collaborative relationships with advocacy groups; actively listening to what such groups have to say; tapping into their ideas and exploring the possible ways in which they could help shape and support the work of researchers makes utter sense. Yet it is not happening on any meaningful scale, despite the phenomenal work that is being done by advocacy groups such as the Multiple Myeloma Research Foundation. In an interview, Leaf summarised just some of the ways in which that potential could be harnessed. He argues that advocacy groups are not simply there to raise monies. A crucial role that such groups could play is in supporting the recruitment process for clinical trials and indeed shaping those trials in fundamental ways.

Leaf's overall assessment is a fierce indictment of a flawed system. However, he also points out that what is broken can be fixed and suggests a viable way forward. He acknowledges that transforming cancer culture will not be easy as the existing culture is so entrenched. Yet, the human cost of allowing things to continue as is, is far too high. His vision of a transformed cancer culture is clear and his arguments are persuasive. The starting point is honesty about data and the complexity of treating such a heterogeneous disease. In Leaf's brave new world, the multiple layers of decision-makers in cancer research would be pared back. The prevailing mindset that the answer always lies in more monies for research would be forever changed. Instead, an effective management system would shake up a culture of caution and align research with the right goals, funding people not projects. He outlines the possibility of creating a collaborative, innovative, coordinated and dynamic global cancer community with a common language and research infrastructure. Radical thinking and creative ideas would be freed up. Most importantly, both ends of the cancer story would be tackled, namely preventing cancer before it strikes and when it does, intervening early and stopping metastasis. His evaluation is shared by many cancer leaders and his views are echoed in later pivotal works such as *The First Cell* by the oncologist Azra Raza. Sadly, the transformative change called for has not happened in the ten years plus since his book first appeared. In a recent *Fortune* magazine article, Leaf considered how the global collaboration that produced Covid vaccines could be tapped into and applied to the world of cancer and might finally kick-start structural change.

Leaf has garnered praise from readers, patient advocacy groups and cancer leaders across America and Europe. For everyone touched by cancer and struggling to see beyond the relentlessly positive spin about advances and breakthroughs, and the constant refrain that a war is being won despite the evidence to the contrary, *The Truth in Small Doses* is a fascinating and absolutely essential read. We can only hope that his message continues to reverberate, with many more figures adding their voices to the call for transformative change. After all, many of our lives, and indeed the lives of future generations, depend on it.

The Immortal Life
of Henrietta Lacks (2010)

Rebecca Skloot
(American writer. Born 1972)

The profoundly unjust nature of cancer care in our world is deeply disturbing. For people whose countries offer universal health coverage, and for people elsewhere with the financial means to access quality health care, the cancer experience is still life threatening and challenging. Simply by accident of birth however, large swathes of the world's population with cancer suffer horribly and have little if any chance of survival, with dire ramifications for individuals, vulnerable families and communities. We are all demeaned by a reality that allows the weak and vulnerable to be ignored, neglected, mistreated and exploited. I dare to believe that cancer experiences can be transformed, but only when equity and human rights take their rightful place at the heart of global health care and medical science. The capacity for change exists. Global activism on the Climate Crisis and the rise of the Black Lives Matter movement give reason for hope. Both movements suggest that people power can be a driver for change nationally and globally. It all begins with opening our minds and our hearts, recognising injustice, refusing to accept it, and then finding effective ways to challenge and pressurise politicians into action. The transformative potential of great storytelling and its capacity to play a role in the battle for social justice should never be underestimated. The question for me was what exceptional book bears witness to cancer's catastrophic impact on the marginalised? What writer has the power to change how the reader sees the injustices that vulnerable people dealing with cancer face? What work prompts readers to see cancer care as a universal human right?

I was reluctant initially to select Skloot's *The Immortal Life of Henrietta Lacks* to fill this niche. After all, it is a widely translated world bestseller, familiar to so many readers and certainly not without flaw. And yet, Skloot's book is also an extraordinary exposé of racial and class injustice, sensitively told. It is a story that matters, giving voice to a family and a community that has been exploited and marginalised for generations. At its heart lies a chilling account of the cervical cancer experience of a thirty-one-year-old African American woman named Henrietta Lacks, and the disastrous consequences for her children of her death. Simultaneously, Skloot chronicles the fascinating history of Henrietta's cancer cells which became the first line of human cells successfully cultured. Named the HeLa line, her cells not only survived but flourished, thus enabling an astonishing range of medical and scientific advances that continues right to the present day.

The injustices suffered by Henrietta's family were compounded when the family were deprived for decades of any knowledge of the existence of the HeLa cell line. Then, when Henrietta's identity became public, the family's privacy was repeatedly violated. Skloot's storytelling ability is matched by both her investigative journalistic skills and her dogged determination to tell what turns out to be a complicated story. The heroic efforts of visionary and committed scientists and doctors are juxtaposed with the darker, exploitative and inhuman face of medicine and science. The tangled web of ethical issues raised by Henrietta's immortal cells is explored. Finally, Skloot reveals the complicated mix of superstition, religion, suspicion and educational disadvantage that has resulted in a distrust of science in America. Anti-science sensibility is now a dominant and lethal force across the world. What is more, it is a force that is vulnerable to manipulation and exploitation. Any hope of dealing with it begins with understanding its roots. This is just one of the many interesting strands woven through Skloot's book. Ultimately, *The Immortal Life of Henrietta Lacks* is essential reading for those of us who dare to hope for a more equitable world where everyone, regardless of race, class or geographic location, has timely access to quality cancer care and is empowered to make informed decisions about treatment choices.

As a cancer biography, Skloot's work makes for harrowing reading, but the facts of Henrietta's short life before her cancer diagnosis are equally bleak. Born into crippling poverty in 1920, Henrietta Lacks lost her mother early and was raised in her grandfather's cabin in Virginia. Her childhood was spent working in the same tobacco fields worked by her slave ancestors. She gave birth to her first child aged fourteen, having shared a bedroom from early childhood with a first cousin whom she married aged twenty. Her cousin infected her with syphilis, and her second child, Elsie, was born with major disabilities as a result. Henrietta first became aware of worrying symptoms during her fifth pregnancy, at a time when she was struggling to meet Elsie's growing needs. On doctor's advice, Elsie was institutionalised. Through Skloot's painstaking research the real woman behind these stark facts emerges. Henrietta was a vibrant, loving, generous-hearted and beautiful woman who embraced life. She loved to cook and to dance, and took pride in her appearance. She also dealt courageously with the many obstacles that crossed her path. Loved by her extended family and friends, she was described as "having a way with children" and planned on having more of her own. She visited Elsie every week without fail until just before her own death and her cousins believed that the loss of Elsie broke her heart. Following the birth of her last son, her symptoms worsened and she was referred to Johns Hopkins, the only hospital for miles that treated African American patients. This marked the start of a brutal cancer experience.

Diagnosed with cervical cancer in February 1951, it is said that she received the best standard treatment of that time although, as Skloot points out, there is no way of knowing for sure. Keeping her diagnosis secret at first, she underwent two radium treatments and never complained of side effects. However, the radiation therapy that followed proved ferocious. As her cancer rapidly spread, exacerbated by syphilis and gonorrhoea, her doctors increased her dose of radiation daily but continued to treat her on an out-patient basis despite her pain.

> When Day (her husband) and the cousins walked home from Sparrows Point after each shift, they could hear Henrietta from a block away, wailing for the Lord to help her.

Henrietta finally pleaded to be admitted to hospital and was placed on a segregated ward in August 1951. Do race and poverty explain the many injustices suffered by Henrietta and her family as treatment progressed or could it simply have been the norm for all patients? In the pre-civil rights era, systemic racism operated unchecked across all areas of society including healthcare. Skloot states:

Several studies have shown that Black patients were treated and hospitalised at later stages of their illnesses than white patients. And once hospitalised, they got fewer pain meds, and had higher mortality rates.

Henrietta's treatment certainly took just such a damning route. The evidence builds that she and her family were never accorded the dignity, respect or compassion that every human being deserves. Her cells were taken during her first radium treatment without her knowledge or consent. Admittedly, this was standard practice at that time. However, by 1951 it was also standard practice to inform patients that infertility was a side-effect of cervical cancer treatment, yet Henrietta was never told. Her concerns about worsening symptoms appear to have been downplayed, if not ignored. When the medical evidence indicated that there was no longer any hope of a cure and treatment became palliative, no one thought to explain this to her family. They continued to believe that doctors were working to cure her and so continued to hope for recovery. Faced with such an aggressive and uncontrollable cancer, radiation treatment finally ceased and in her medical record Henrietta was then referred to as "a miserable specimen" who "groans". Blood transfusions were also stopped until her financial deficit with the blood bank was made up. The final image of Henrietta, suffering unrelenting waves of pain, is haunting. In the absence of effective pain relief, her limbs were strapped down to stop her thrashing about and a pillow was thrust into her mouth to stop her biting her tongue. Henrietta died in October 1951 aged just thirty-one and was buried in an unmarked grave, seemingly destined to fade quickly from history. And yet her legacy had already begun to change the world of science through the work of the visionary cell biologist George Gey.

In the Johns Hopkins cancer research lab, Gey and his wife, Margaret, a surgical nurse, had been struggling and failing to create a cell line for decades. As head of tissue research, George Gey was given Henrietta's cervical cancer tissue. Using self-developed techniques and instruments, and adhering to Margaret's strict sterility rules, he finally made the breakthrough long strived for, establishing the first line of human cells that survived and thrived outside the body. Driven by a fierce desire for scientific advancement, he also developed effective methods to transport HeLa cells and began sharing them with scientists around the world. In so doing, he helped revolutionise scientific research across many fields. Three Nobel Prizes to date have been awarded to scientists whose discoveries rest on studies in the HeLa cell line. HeLa cells helped launch the field of virology and played a central role in the eradication of polio, the development of HPV vaccines and the testing of HIV drugs. Indeed, HeLa most recently helped pave the way for Covid-19 research breakthroughs. Advances in IVF and cloning rest on research using the HeLa line. The contribution made to cancer research is no less impressive. Chemotherapy drugs, gene mapping and diagnostic tests have been evaluated or developed using HeLa. The FISH test is a perfect example. Best known for its role in the field of breast cancer, it is also critical for the care of patients with chronic lymphocytic leukaemia. I am therefore just one of the countless millions who owe a debt of gratitude to Henrietta and to the scientists who have delivered major breakthroughs using her cultured cells. Unquestionably, George and Margaret Gey are heroic figures who never exploited HeLa's commercial potential. However, with demand for the HeLa cell line growing exponentially, a multibillion dollar industry selling HeLa cells and other human material was born. It raised complex ethical issues about ownership, informed consent, trust and compensation. Scientific careers and reputations were not the only thing that flourished because of HeLa. Financial fortunes were made. Yet Henrietta's family continued to live in poverty. Henrietta's daughter Deborah captured the irony of this state of affairs:

> "But I always thought it was strange, if our mother's cells done so much for medicine, how come her family can't afford to see no doctors? Don't make no sense."

When Gey died in 1970, an article published in his honour outlined the HeLa cell line's history and contained Henrietta's full name and her photographic image. News of Henrietta's immortal cells spread quickly and eventually reached the family for the first time. To fully understand their response, Skloot traces the family history following the death of Henrietta, focusing most especially on Deborah with whom she developed a close relationship as she helped her uncover the true story of Deborah's mother, her sister Elsie, and the HeLa cells.

The impact of Henrietta's death on her children's lives was nothing less than catastrophic. They were not even told of their mother's death – it was as if Henrietta had suddenly just disappeared, never to be spoken of again. Left in the care of an abusive couple, their subsequent childhood was marked by hunger, vicious beatings and enforced work. Joe, the youngest, who was just a baby when Henrietta died, seems to have borne the brunt of the violence. Deborah endured years of sexual as well as physical abuse. The scars of their blighted childhood and bitter experiences were carried into their adult lives which were marked by poverty, ill health, spousal abuse, delinquency and violence. The fate of their institutionalised sister Elsie was even grimmer. She was never visited after Henrietta's death and she died aged 15, before Deborah even learned of her existence. The monstrosity of what transpired in Crownsville State Hospital, where Elsie was housed, is exposed. Conditions were even worse than those experienced in Irish industrial schools or Ceausescu's orphanages. Elsie was subjected to squalor, gross overcrowding, abuse and horrifying medical experimentation. Skloot describes a sinister photograph found in an official file of a terrified Elsie bearing facial injuries and with a "large pair of white hands" forcefully holding her face to camera. It powerfully conveys the level of depravity and the culpability of state authorities who allowed it to happen. Antonia Hylton's meticulously researched 2024 book *Madness: Race and Insanity in America* corroborates Skloot's account of Crownsville. When racism, poverty, misogyny and disability combine, the perfect dehumanising storm results.

An arduous emotional ordeal began for the family upon learning of the existence of Henrietta's immortal cells. It would continue for decades as scientists and journalists repeatedly violated their trust and their privacy whilst utterly failing to help them understand the science behind HeLa. Blood samples were taken for research purposes without proper explanation. Family genetic information was subsequently published without their consent. Henrietta's medical records were released and then extensively quoted in a book about HeLa without prior family approval. When they learnt from a 1976 *Rolling Stone* article about the money being generated from HeLa sales, Henrietta's sons became convinced that George Gey and Johns Hopkins had stolen Henrietta's cells and made a fortune from them. They fixated on this so-called injustice for years. Meanwhile, Deborah struggled to understand the science and discover the truth about her mother. She bombarded every journalist and scientist she encountered with questions but was ill-equipped to understand their explanations. The family was hampered by educational disadvantage and a deep-seated distrust of science. No doubt the long history of medical abuse of African Americans, carried out with impunity, played its part in building such distrust. The family was also embittered by years of exploitation and understandably suspicious of the motives of those who sought them out because of HeLa. They were by turns enraged, confused and terrified for decades and the toll on the family was huge. It is to Skloot's credit that she persevered with the story, patiently building a rocky but ultimately healing relationship with Deborah. Skloot committed a decade of her life to helping Deborah uncover and understand the truth of Henrietta's life, her death and her immortal cells. In the most moving chapter, Skloot accompanies Deborah and her deeply troubled brother Zakhariyya to Johns Hopkins at the invitation of PhD student Christoph Lengauer. It is a cathartic moment. Finally, they "meet" their mother, hold a HeLa test tube in their hands and view her cells under a microscope. Lengauer's frank admission that the hospital had screwed up and his determination to give them all the time and support they needed was momentous. Deborah and her brother responded with grace. Yet the reader cannot fail to notice that the family was only accorded the respect and dignity they deserved fifty years after Henrietta's death and nearly thirty years after they first learned of Henrietta's immortal cells.

> As we walked toward the elevator, Zakhariyya reached up and touched Christoph on the back and said thank you. Outside, he did the same to me, then turned to catch the bus home. Deb and I stood in silence, watching him walk away. Then she put her arm around me and said, "Girl, you just witnessed a miracle."

The wonder and pride of the Lacks family in Henrietta's immense contribution to medicine and science is well founded. Their desire to see the HeLa line continue to serve scientific research whilst also being properly acknowledged reflects their generosity of spirit.

Skloot exposes the complex ethical issues surrounding cancer research. She raises awareness of the need for effective laws and policing mechanisms that keep pace with scientific advances and safeguard patient rights. In telling the story of the Lacks family's long and bitter experiences and demeaning treatment, she opens our eyes to the long-term devastating impacts of injustice. There is a moral imperative to *The Immortal Life of Henrietta Lacks* that is inescapable. This dense and complicated story is a clarion call for equity and human rights to be placed at the heart of health care provision. A world in which every cancer patient has timely access to quality cancer services without financial worries and is cared for with compassion and respect is a world worth hoping and fighting for. If Skloot's vivid portrait of Henrietta and her family plays a part in altering how people see injustice, and more specifically health injustice, it could just prove to be as transformational as Henrietta's immortal cells.

Reading and Writing Cancer: How Words Heal (2016)

Susan Gubar

(*American writer. Born 1944*)

Could *Reading and Writing Cancer* be the book that I had longed for on diagnosis, searched for to no avail for years, and consequently set out to write for myself? If so, then my years of research and writing would be redundant. Happily, although Gubar shares my belief in the power of the written word to heal, her approach in *Reading and Writing Cancer* is quite different from, although complementary to, my own. Gubar offers the reader an alternative route into the world of cancer literature. By addressing those living with cancer who want to write about the impact of the disease, and those who want to engage with cancer literature through extensive reading, Gubar sees her book as serving a dual purpose.

> I have sought to create a mix between a manual and a map: a manual for those who want to write, a map for those who want to read.

It would be hard to find a more qualified person to deliver on that aim. Susan Gubar is a renowned literary author, feminist and academic. Diagnosed with late-stage BRCA-related ovarian cancer in 2008, she underwent multiple radical surgeries, chemotherapy cycles and radiological procedures, before entering a clinical trial for the experimental Pfizer drug that saved her life.

Gubar's dedication to literature continued, albeit with her professional eye now trained on a new and urgent subject, that is reading and writing about cancer. The year 2012 proved to be transformative on three counts. She entered the clinical trial that saved her life; published her starkly honest and moving book *Memoir of a Debulked Woman: Enduring Ovarian Cancer*, and began writing a monthly column, 'Living With Cancer', for the *New York Times*. Gubar has mastered the art of opinion writing. Her engaging style is married with a wealth of knowledge and experience of living with cancer. She has also developed a journalist's unerring eye for what matters to the reader. A recent column about the perils of being dependent for your survival on a clinical trial for access to lifesaving, outrageously expensive drugs is a case in point. In *Reading & Writing Cancer*, Gubar brings all of these skills to deliver a book that will energise and enthuse readers interested in the healing benefits of dealing with cancer through the written word. As is to be expected from an academic, Gubar's book is well structured, with four themed chapters and a preface that outlines exactly what is contained in each section and why. Wisely, she concludes with an extensive 'Notes and Suggested Readings' section that is a launch pad for those who want to venture deeper into the world of cancer literature.

For Gubar, the act of writing has proven to be a lifeline and her focus in two of the four chapters is on helping those who want to write effectively. She starts the writing cancer half of her book by making a compelling case for writing as a "restorative activity" and a vital means of grappling with the impact of cancer. Using her experience as author, blogger and cancer patient, and supported by evidence garnered from the research and insight of sociologists, psychologists and writers, she postulates that:

> The writing process enables a reconstitution of the self ... Be it angry or sorrowful, defiant or resigned, courageous or fearful, this emergent voice helps us understand who we are becoming ... Even and perhaps especially during times of loss, we may need to urge ourselves to '*Write*' it. For writing provides a way not necessarily to master disaster, but to comprehend and accept or contend with it ... While writing, we become less sick or debilitated because we are conceptualising how it feels or what it means to be sick or debilitated.

Gubar highlights how writing is a perfect fit for cancer patients forced by serious illness into a restrictive and often isolated life. She points out its many advantages for the cancer patient. It is a sedentary, solitary and cheap activity that can be undertaken anywhere, requiring only the simplest of tools. It can be done in short spurts or in longer blocks of time, picked up or dropped at a moment's notice. At the very time when cancer patients are forced to relinquish control over so many aspects of their lives to medical specialists and carers, the act of writing – in sharp contrast – empowers. The writer has total control over every word on the page, time can be suspended during composition and something truly meaningful achieved if the skills of writing are developed. Gubar has no doubt that this is achievable and sets out to show us how.

Ideas, exercises and prompts are offered to stimulate and develop the writing habit. She stresses the importance of reading widely and paying close attention to the techniques and styles of eminent writers. The creative challenges of free writing, expressive writing, journaling and memoir writing are considered. Gubar devotes one chapter solely to blogging, appreciating how it can work well for the cancer patient. Using her personal experience, she explores the blog's potential, its strengths and limitations, and the ethical issues it raises. The opportunities a blog gives a writer to address personal fears and concerns, explore difficult experiences, reach a large audience and even take on a patient advocacy role are detailed. However, Gubar does not shy away from the flip side of blogging, summarising it well in a comment about how a blog's immediacy and limitless reach "can breed exhibitionism in writers, while provoking voyeurism in readers". As challenging and satisfying as Gubar has clearly found her blog to be, one thought on the subject is telling:

> Paradoxically, though, the blog has convinced me of the virtues of the printed book.

Informed by her own experience of serious illness, what Gubar has to say about writing will help the budding author with cancer. She covers all of the essentials and is clear, insightful, practical and succinct.

Where Gubar's work is unique and undoubtedly shines, however, is in her razor-sharp analysis of reading cancer. Suggested works abound across all chapters but in two – 'Impatient Memoirs' and 'Sublime Artistry' – she positively revels in introducing us to the finest cancer literature. The whole guide is a veritable reading goldmine. It is a testament to the breadth and depth of Gubar's own reading and to her skills as an accomplished literary critic. In tackling cancer memoirs, she puts much-needed shape on this ever-growing genre, tracing its surprisingly long lineage and grouping work by recurring themes and perspectives. Gubar managed to introduce authors and titles new to me, despite my familiarity with the genre. Most pleasing of all was finding some of my chosen memoirs included in her work. Gubar's response to works by Audre Lorde, John Diamond and Christina Wiman mirrored my own views and, in so doing, reassured me that I was right on track. Her final words on cancer memoirs summarise their significance.

> Since cancer and its treatments so often imperil or fracture the self, the genre of memoir – which proposes an individual identity – engages readers by evincing the resiliency of individuals who transmute or transcend their roles as patients ... we can learn to become learners from the angry, fearful, funny, satiric, and exceptionally patient memoirists whose publications help us understand how to become our unbecoming selves.

In the chapter 'Sublime Artistry', Gubar turns to literary fiction and the visual arts to make sense of the cancer experience and deepen understanding of life and death. She sets out to prove how great literature can heal the scars that cancer leaves on "the psyche, the soul, the spirit". Her reflections on an extensive range of novels and short stories are candid, striking and keenly perceptive. Although Gubar is an academic, there is nothing at all intimidating about her approach for the general reader. In fact, Gubar's words cannot fail to enthuse, encouraging a return to old favourites and a desire to read newly discovered voices. Once again, I was pleased to find that Gubar shared my appreciation for key works in the cancer canon. I enjoyed her unique take on novels, novellas and short stories. Encapsulating her thoughts on the power of creative works about cancer she states:

> That we are looking at or reading about suffering in highly crafted forms reassures us that we can gain insight into the travails we ourselves may have to face ... Creative thinkers seek – often in experimental or shorter forms – to wrest meaning from suffering.

I must admit that Gubar's consideration of visual art and graphic novels went largely over my head but no doubt these areas are of great interest to other readers. What was surprising and perplexing was her decision to exclude an insightful tour of cancer poetry to equal her enlightening surveys of other literary genres. Her reasoning for this exclusion is outlined.

> I also felt and still believe that this poetic tradition is only now emerging and that I do not have sufficient acumen to choose one text or another as more representative than any other.

While shying away from poetry analysis, Gubar does piece together a cancer cento from the work of twenty poets and recommends that the reader follow up by searching for their work. Although the cento is clever and the references are welcome, I was more than a little disappointed by this approach, especially given Gubar's critical powers and her previous publishing history. The absence of poetry from *Reading and Writing Cancer* could have led me to question my decision to include poetry in this work. In fact, it only strengthened my resolve as I now regard poetry as first among equals in articulating cancer experiences. Interestingly, when Gubar searched for a powerful way to close her book with words that "reflect my conviction that reading and writing have an amazing capacity to buoy hale spirits in frail bodies", it is to poetry that she turns, more specifically to Raymond Carver's glorious poem 'Gravy'.

Despite these small reservations, *Reading & Writing Cancer* is a book worth seeking out. It is an invigorating read, written by a woman with an in-depth knowledge of literature and a willingness to mine her own difficult cancer experiences to help others. Her arguments for the healing power of literature convince. Her passion for words that heal is infectious. Fledgling writers will find her practical advice useful as they set out to capture in words their own cancer experience. In the end, though, it is Gubar's skilful exploration of the world of cancer literature, carried out with zeal and covering a wealth of the finest writing, that proves utterly irresistible. Gubar has indeed created a wonderful map of the cancer canon. She has accomplished something that is of real benefit for readers living and dying with cancer and searching for consolation.

A Grief Observed (1961)

C. S. Lewis

(Irish writer 1898–1963)

In my search for literature that captures fundamental truths about the continuum of devastating losses that is the cancer experience, I found myself constantly drawn back to *A Grief Observed*. Revered as a classic of grief literature, it is a compelling account of one man's experience of bereavement. It is also a powerful interrogation of aspects of loss, love, suffering, religious faith and death that trouble many of us struggling with cancer. In writing it, the reader senses that Lewis was not simply grappling with his own personal demons but consciously reaching out to connect with others trapped in an abyss of agony, rage and despair. Lewis's analytical mind, intellectual force, writer's sensibility and above all his humanity, come together in perfect union in this short book, throwing light onto our most feared existential conundrums. Questions pour out but many prove unanswerable. It is such a relief to read his words precisely because he reaches no tidy resolutions and delivers no pat answers. Instead, we get a lucid, coherent and intense portrait of a suffering mind that is searching for and slowly finding a path back to life.

    Born in Belfast, Lewis was educated in England from the age of nine. Over a lifelong academic career in Oxford and latterly in Cambridge, he flourished as an enormously popular and inspiring lecturer and as a scholarly writer. One of a generation shaped by First World War experiences, it is little wonder that Lewis's fictional output reflects a preoccupation with the battle between good and evil. An atheist from his teenage years, he returned to his Christian faith in the early 1930s and became a hugely influential Christian writer. Lewis's series of radio broadcasts on Christian faith during the Second World War attracted large audiences, received critical acclaim and made him a household name. Subsequently, these broadcasts were anthologised in a book entitled *Mere Christianity*. Regarded as a classic defence of the Christian faith, it is consistently ranked as one of the most influential religious books of the 20th century and continues to be widely read. *Mere Christianity* is eclipsed, however, by the massive popularity of his beloved Chronicles of Narnia. This classic series of seven children's allegorical novels has retained its hold on the imaginations of generations of children and adults alike across the world. Narnia showcases Lewis's storytelling skills but also his fondness for exploring the meaning of life imaginatively. Widely considered to be a quintessential Englishman, the publication of his personal correspondence in recent years has only confirmed what many long suspected. His Irish background and love for Irish mythology, Hiberno-English and the landscape of Ireland heavily influenced his life and his writing. Aware of the sectarian nature of his home place and repelled by bigotry and colonial violence, Lewis took an ecumenical stance in his Christian faith. He saw himself as Irish and was seen by his friends and colleagues as Irish, so is included in this work as an Irish writer.

The two great tragedies of Lewis's life were caused by cancer. The loss of his mother when he was just nine years old shattered his world. Her death reverberated throughout his life and its impact can be seen in his fiction. The loss of his wife sparked a grief that remained raw to the end of his life. Lewis's rage and sense of powerlessness is palpable from the outset of *A Grief Observed*.

Cancer, and cancer, and cancer. My mother, my father, my wife.
I wonder who is next in the queue.

The backstory of Lewis's relationship with the American poet Joy Davidman is no doubt familiar to many. Their relationship began in 1950 when Davidman first wrote to Lewis. A regular correspondence developed that centred on literature and theology. In 1952 they met face to face for the first time. Following the break-up of Davidman's first marriage and her subsequent move to England with her two sons, the friendship deepened. When immigration issues arose in 1956, Lewis and Davidman married in a civil ceremony that was seen by Lewis as purely a matter of "friendship and expediency". They continued to live separately until Davidman was diagnosed with advanced and incurable metastatic cancer. This shock brought Lewis to the realisation that he was deeply in love. A second but this time religious marriage ceremony took place at Davidman's hospital bedside. Subsequent treatment resulted in remission and they had three intensely happy years in which to relish their late-flowering love. However, cancer recurred and Davidman died in July 1960. *A Grief Observed* was written as an immediate response to this crushing loss and was first published under the pseudonym N.W. Clerk, not appearing under Lewis's own name until after his death.

Lewis places the vivid presence of Davidman, referred to throughout as "H", centre stage in *A Grief Observed*. With every reference to "H" and to their relationship we notice afresh just how open and personal *A Grief Observed* is. Lewis is trusting the reader with his most intimate thoughts and emotions. There is no mistaking Lewis's admiration for his wife nor the annihilating nature of his loss. Lewis's great fear is of forgetting her. Perhaps even worse, he dreads reshaping her over time in his memory, thereby obscuring, distorting and eventually losing sight of the real woman. Some of the last letters he ever wrote testify to how raw and enduring his sense of loss was.

In giving his personal perspective on grief, Lewis also captures so many universal aspects of what it is to live with traumatic loss of any kind. The opening lines of *A Grief Observed* plunge us straight into his shattered mind. Beset by fear, confusion, despair, self-pity, isolation, and a sense of unreality, he is trapped in distorted time. Nothing makes sense anymore. Emotionally paralysed, he finds it impossible to care about anything. Moments arise when memories flood back and the agony of loss torments him yet again. Thoughts swirl uncontrollably and endlessly. He struggles to figure out how to process his loss and so re-discover meaning in life and in love. Even in the midst of grief, Lewis is still the same lucid thinker and writer of compulsively readable prose, consciously reaching out to the reader.

> Aren't all these notes the senseless writhings of a man who won't accept the fact that there is nothing we can do with suffering except to suffer it? Who still thinks there is some device (if only he could find it) which will make pain not to be pain … And grief still feels like fear. Perhaps, more strictly, like suspense … It gives life a permanently provisional feeling … Up till this I always had too little time. Now there is nothing but time. Almost pure time, empty successiveness.

Lewis's love for Davidman was an integral part of a greater love, that is his love of God. We are left in no doubt that the loss of the person Lewis loved so intensely has obliterated his entire world and shaken to the core his sense of self and his faith in a merciful God. He finds himself in crisis, with the old certainties that he so confidently held now turned into vexed questions that must be grappled with. Lewis refuses to evade such fears and doubts, choosing instead to face the questions that grievous loss has raised. As *A Grief Observed* progresses, it becomes an exploration of a faith racked by doubt. To go to God when most in need only to find that he is nowhere to be found horrifies him and triggers fury.

His sense of betrayal is powerfully described through an experience all too familiar to those on cancer's rollercoaster, hoping and praying like Lewis for a return to stable ground. When potential exits prove to be a mirage and no help seems forthcoming, fear grows that God is absent, uncaring, cruel or even non-existent, and the only reality is further suffering.

> What chokes every prayer and every hope is the memory of all the prayers H and I offered and all the false hopes we had. Not hopes raised merely by our own wishful thinking; hopes encouraged, even forced upon us, by false diagnoses, by X-ray photographs, by strange remissions, by one temporary recovery that might have ranked as a miracle. Step by step we were 'led up the garden path'. Time after time, when He seemed most gracious He was really preparing the next torture.

For Lewis, it is never really a question of whether God exists. His faith is sorely tested but its framework holds firm. He continues to see through a Christian lens. The question that bedevils him is, if God is good, how can he allow such terrible suffering? He gradually reaches a standpoint on this difficult issue and presents it to us by way of a typically rational and direct question.

> But is it credible that such extremities of torture should be necessary for us? Well, take your choice. The tortures occur. If they are unnecessary, then there is no God or a bad one. If there is a good God, then these tortures are necessary.

We see where Lewis's thinking is leading him and what his answer to that question is. He is moving back to faith in a loving God and understanding more about what blocks his path. Ever conscious of his human frailty, he compares his faith to a house of cards that has been knocked down by adversity and remains perpetually vulnerable to doubt.

Lewis fleshes out the insights that interrogation of his experience with loss has revealed. His hard-earned wisdom can be summarised as follows: profound loss is an integral and universal part of living and of loving. We need to become reconciled to the reality that grieving is a natural response to loss and is an agonising, complex process without a timetable. We must learn to accept that sometimes there really are no answers and acknowledge that there is so much that we can never understand. There is purpose in human suffering even if we cannot discern it. One purpose, Lewis believes, lies in how suffering breaks down our simplistic ideas of God and forces us to reshape our faith. Lewis's description of the 'gains' won from such an intense examination of his grief is characteristically understated yet also heavy with meaning.

A Grief Observed speaks with scrupulous honesty and clarity to every human heart in crisis. This exceptional, concise book can help believers and non-believers alike make sense of, and come to terms with, the complex and topsy-turvy nature of suffering. There is no mistaking the parallels with Donald Hall's book *Without*. Both writers wailed the loss of their beloved wives in the written word, and mourned them for the rest of their lives. Hall's poetry about Jane seems to echo Lewis's prose about Joy. Given how influential *A Grief Observed* has been from its first appearance in print, I like to imagine that Hall was consoled by what Lewis has to say about such grievous loss.

Of the two convictions that Lewis puts forward in his closing pages, I choose to carry with me the hopeful and consoling one. Quoting the Christian mystic Julian of Norwich, Lewis states:

… and all shall be well, and all manner of thing shall be well.

Gratitude (2015)

Oliver Sacks

(*English writer 1933–2015*)

My generation was lucky enough to reap the benefits of the work of Irish feminists who, from the early 1970s on, challenged and changed Irish society. The leaders of that movement, many of whom were outstanding journalists, were my earliest heroes. Even amongst such illustrious company, Nuala O'Faolain always stood out. Her opinion column in the *Irish Times* was witty, authoritative and perceptive. She had a knack for getting to the crux of whatever topic caught her attention and the ability to convey that essence to readers. I recall reading aloud one of her opinion pieces – a perfectly judged and wonderfully moving column about adult literacy – at a celebratory event in Cavan library to a rapturous response from adult learners. They recognised and appreciated the truth and beauty of O'Faolain's piece. Throughout the 1980s and 1990s O'Faolain continued to break the deafening silence around a diverse range of taboo subjects as her journalistic career unfolded. When her memoir *Are You Somebody?* was published, to justified acclaim, I witnessed at first hand the remarkable connection she had established with her readers over the course of a magical and intimate evening in Crannóg, Cavan's great bookshop, now sadly gone.

O'Faolain's speaking voice was as instantly recognisable as her authorial voice. Hearing that distinctive voice on radio was an immediate prompt to listen attentively. Over the winter of 2007–2008 I eagerly listened out for her regular slot on Mary Wilson's *Drivetime* radio show. Her coverage of the U.S.

Democratic Party Presidential Primaries was superb. The drama unfolding between Obama and Clinton left many feminists conflicted – but not Nuala. She recognised the historical significance of the nomination of a woman but also accurately observed that Clinton would in all likelihood fail to secure the nomination. Without warning and much to my chagrin, Nuala's slot simply disappeared and I waited impatiently for its return. I could never have anticipated just how riveting Nuala's next interview on radio would prove to be.

On April 12th, 2008, on Marian Finucane's Saturday morning radio show, O'Faolain revealed that she had been diagnosed with an incurable cancer just six weeks previously, had received radiation treatment but had decided against undergoing chemotherapy, and was now dying. Like so many listeners, I was shocked and saddened to learn that this unique and gifted woman, who had made such an enormous contribution to Irish public and literary life, was to be lost to us. The facts were brutal enough, but it was the anger and despair in her voice that was truly heart-breaking. With the searing honesty that had always been her trademark she revealed the depth of her anguish. The words she used so eloquently are scorched into my memory. Cancer "reduced me to impotence and wretchedness". She spoke of how, on hearing her bleak prognosis, life had quickly turned black with all the goodness gone. The joy she had found in many things, including literature, drained away and all that remained were "sourness and fear". She nailed a reality all too familiar to those living and dying with cancer when she stated that "the very essence of this experience is aloneness". Nuala sounded utterly inconsolable and devoid of hope. Of the many feelings expressed, one in particular horrified me. She spoke about what a waste of creation life is when, with each death, all that knowledge dies. For Nuala, in that moment, death meant non-existence and therefore life had no meaning. The self-doubt that had always plagued her seemed to have blinded her not only to how meaningful and worthwhile her life had been but also to her important legacy.

Looking back, I believe that the seed of an idea was planted at that very moment although it didn't start to bloom until many years later. I was convinced that somewhere in the world of literature there was a perfect piece of prose or poetry that had the power to help Nuala discern how truly meaningful her life was. It would provide her, and indeed anyone whose spirit was being annihilated by cancer, with some measure of peace and consolation as death approached. If I researched earnestly, I was convinced that I would find such a work. When I came across the remarkable book *Gratitude,* I knew that my search was over.

My first encounter with the neurologist and writer Oliver Sacks arose out of my work as Cavan Co. Librarian. In the early 2000s, a determination to make the Central Library, then under construction, universally accessible required consultation with local people with disabilities. I intuitively understood that consultation would only be truly effective if I had a real grasp of what it is like to be amongst the most excluded members of society. So, as a starting point, I immersed myself in the literature of disability and soon stumbled upon two extraordinary books by Oliver Sacks: *Seeing Voices* and *Awakenings*. This gifted writer and storyteller brought case histories to life, shining a light on each patient's unique abilities, vulnerabilities, challenges and resilience. A sensitive and empathetic doctor, he used his brilliant mind and wide-ranging scientific and medical knowledge to help people who were institutionalised, largely ignored and often abandoned by wider society. Although Oliver Sacks provoked criticism from some disability rights activists and commentators who suggested that he objectified patients and reinforced medical power, his body of work gives the lie to such assertions. His work is in fact rooted in a desire to heal and radiates sensitivity, tact, respect and understanding. Paul Theroux's memorable profile of Oliver Sacks in his recent essay collection, *Figures in a Landscape*, captures the essence of this erudite, generous and compassionate man who blazed a trail in medicine, science and literature.

Oliver Sacks was a complex and eccentric genius shaped by tough life experiences. In a string of books, including two outstanding memoirs, he chronicled critical turning points in his own life. The child abuse he endured for years after his evacuation from London during the Blitz embedded a sense of fear, dislocation and insecurity in his psyche. Growing up with a schizophrenic brother whose medical care was grossly mismanaged, and whom he was terrified for but also desperate to escape from, helped shape his career direction. His mother's cruel rejection and the feelings of shame that she engendered on learning that he was homosexual scarred him. It triggered a move to Canada and then onwards to America and no doubt contributed to his descent into a drug addiction that nearly killed him. With the help of an analyst, Sacks built a slow recovery from his self-destructive impulses, including his drug addiction. He retreated into a solitary and celibate life, kept his sexuality a closely guarded secret for years and focused on his two primary passions – writing and neurology. Acutely sensitive to the patient's perspective, he gained fresh insight into the world of illness from his personal experience of sickness and frailty which included a serious hiking accident, a cancer diagnosis and a lifelong cognitive disorder known as prosopagnosia (face blindness). His understanding of how serious illness fundamentally changes people permeates much of his writing, as does his intellectual curiosity, optimistic tone and unwavering enthusiasm for life.

In addition to writing books, Sacks was a prolific essayist and his wide-ranging articles and essays attest to his ability to move fluidly across disciplines. Four essays written in the last two years of his life are an extraordinary gift for those of us living and dying with cancer. Initially published separately in the *New York Times*, this quartet of essays was published together posthumously in a beautifully produced book, aptly titled *Gratitude*. A slim work, just forty-five pages long, it is dense with meaning and truth. Sacks gives what one reviewer fittingly calls "a statement of departure". It is a clear-eyed meditation on life, on serious illness, and on using the time of dying to take stock but also to live as productively and intensely as possible as life's final challenge is faced. It is a book to be treasured, read and returned to time and again. Imbued with serenity and gratitude, it has such power to heal that the title *Solace* would be equally appropriate.

Gratitude is a beautiful object and a pure pleasure to hold, a printed work that is a sensory delight. Relish the feel of its fabric cover. Enjoy the beautiful endpapers with a perfect amount of biographical information and an astute endorsement by Atul Gawande. Just seven carefully selected photographs are perfectly placed within the text and enhance our sense of the author. Within its covers, the content of each essay somehow coalesces into something greater than the sum of its parts. The first essay, *Mercury*, was written just before Sack's eightieth birthday as he considered how he felt about life and ageing. He expresses his deep sense of gratitude for all that has been given to him by others and for all that he has been able to contribute to the world. His passion for life shines in his writing, although he also acknowledges the signs of decline that are an inevitable part of ageing. Sacks's first essay reminded me of Donald Hall's delightfully amusing *Essays After Eighty*. Like Hall, Sacks sees old age as a ceremony of losses but conveys a similar sense of gratitude for life.

> Perhaps, with luck, I will make it, more or less intact, for another few years and be granted the liberty to continue to love and work, the two most important things, Freud insisted, in life.

His positive view of old age reflects the feelings of his father who lived to ninety-four.

He felt, as I begin to feel, not a shrinking but an enlargement of mental life and perspective.

My Own Life, the second essay of the quartet, was written eighteen months later, soon after Sacks learned that a cancer, long in remission, had metastasized and death was now fast approaching. Rather than brooding on his misfortune, he focuses on his gratitude for the nine years of remission that enabled him to live fully and productively. In facing death, he speaks of choosing to live his dying days in "the richest, deepest, most productive way I can" and considers how his perspective on life has subtly shifted.

I have been able to see my life as from a great altitude, as a sort of landscape, and with a deepening sense of the connection of all its parts … I feel intensely alive … I feel a sudden clear focus and perspective. There is no time for anything inessential.

In the final, breath-taking passage of *My Own Life* he encapsulates his view of life.

"I cannot pretend I am without fear. But my predominant feeling is one of gratitude. I have loved and been loved; I have been given much and I have given something in return; I have read and travelled and thought and written. I have had intercourse with the world, the special intercourse of writers and readers.
Above all, I have been a sentient being, a thinking animal, on this beautiful planet, and that in itself has been an enormous privilege and adventure.

The few months of relatively good health that followed treatment, which Sacks refers to as "an intermission", were filled with living: writing, spending time with friends, travelling and immersing himself in the world of science which had been his comfort since childhood. The third essay, *My Periodic Table*, was produced during this period and pays homage to his lifelong love for the periodic table of the elements. He writes of his regret that he will not live to see future scientific breakthroughs and of how, while viewing the grandeur of the night sky, he suddenly realised how little life remains for him.

> My sense of the heavens' beauty, of eternity, was inseparably mixed for me with a sense of transience – and death.

The fourth and final essay, 'Sabbath', is one that Sacks laboured over, and to great effect. Taking stock of his life, he begins with a consideration of the orthodox Jewish traditions of his youth which he cast aside following his mother's rejection of his sexuality. As he delves into the major events of his life and touches on the turning points that shaped him, painful issues are unearthed and considered. Sacks brings his story full circle when he recounts a healing reunion with his deeply religious extended family in Israel. Despite his fears, he and his partner, Bill Hayes, are not simply accepted, but warmly welcomed by the family. With this embrace, his mother's devastating rejection is finally ameliorated. Although Sacks never believed in God or an afterlife, his Jewish identity was of growing concern to him in his dying days and he was drawn to, and comforted by, the practice of Jewish traditions. It is to those traditions that he turns in his deeply moving closing paragraph.

> And now, weak, short of breath, my once-firm muscles melted away by cancer, I find my thoughts, increasingly, not on the supernatural or spiritual but on what is meant by living a good and worthwhile life – achieving a sense of peace within oneself. I find my thoughts drifting to the Sabbath, the day of rest, the seventh day of the week, and perhaps the seventh day of one's life as well, when one can feel that one's work is done, and one may, in good conscience, rest.

There is no finer way of concluding this gathering of treasures than with *Gratitude*. Sacks's book is a wonderful act of solidarity, reminding us that we are not alone in our suffering. His heart speaks articulately and directly to ours, offering precious glimpses of clarity and insight. His compassionate and erudite mind cuts straight to what matters in how we choose to live and how we approach our dying. It seems to me that he is calling on all of us to be committed to living intensely, appreciating every moment of the life that is given to us. Furthermore, he urges us to believe that the act of living has meaning and to work at creating our own sense of peace. The alchemy of reading brings Sacks into our hearts, a literary companion who helps us work out what truly matters. Sadly, *Gratitude* was published more than seven years after Nuala O'Faolain's death and so could not provide her with the solace she so desperately needed.

However, I like to believe that the outpouring of respect, appreciation and love that followed O'Faolain's last interview was a welcome reminder that her life had been a good and useful one, full of meaning, and that some measure of peace and consolation flowed from that knowledge. Sacks expressed the hope that

> ... some of my books may still speak to people after my death.

Nuala O'Faolain's *Are You Somebody* will be read and appreciated for generations to come, as will no doubt Sacks's perfectly formed and remarkable little book. *Gratitude* is chock-full of heart, spirit and wisdom. I wholeheartedly believe that it will be cherished by every reader lucky enough to encounter it.

Sacks's work is the final addition to this lifeline of cancer writing that I am passionate about sharing. For the life-changing experience that is cancer, life-saving writing is indispensable. Coming to terms with overwhelming feelings and existential questions requires strength of spirit. The profound words of every writer honoured in this collection feed that spirit. When we read any one of these works, something changes in our hearts and souls that is forever changed. This is writing that builds our mental and spiritual stamina to cope with the cancer rollercoaster and the consequential loss of control of our lives. It furnishes us with sheltering, reflective places of healing quiet, where the breath of consolation awaits. In so many ways, endurance is the key. Endurance is the enactment of hope. It is hope made possible. With these literary companions by our side, we can endure, we can find meaning, and we can live in hope. Despite the heartache, challenges and losses that cancer brings, we can rediscover the joy of living to the fullest extent possible.

Acknowledgements

My sincere thanks to the inspiring writers
who populate this book and make it a place of sanctuary and solace
for all who suffer because of cancer.

I am grateful to the authors' families, agents, editors
and staff in publishing companies worldwide,
who supported me in clearing permissions.

The international community of librarians ensured that
my quest for information and access to material –
especially during the Covid years – bore fruit.
Thank you.

Without the encouragement of the writers
John Quinn, Brian Keenan, Niall MacMonagle,
Martina Devlin and Dermot Bolger, this book might never
have made it into print. I am forever in your debt.

Extended Copyright

I am grateful to the following for permission to reproduce copyright material:

James Baldwin: From 'James Baldwin Writing and Talking' interview, the *New York Times* 23rd September, 1979. Reproduced by permission of the LLC Rights Agency for the James Baldwin Estate.

Pat Barker: Short story 'Muriel Scaife' from *Union Street*. Published by Virago Press. Copyright © Pat Barker, 1982. Quoted with permission from Pat Barker.

Lucia Berlin: Five short stories from *A Manual for Cleaning Women: Selected Stories*, with a foreword by Lydia Davis. Published by Picador. Copyright © The Estate of Lucia Berlin 2015. Reproduced with permission of Pan Macmillan through PLSclear.

Georgia Blain: From *The Museum of Words: A memoir of language, writing and mortality* and *Between a wolf and a dog*. Copyright © Estate of Georgia Blain 2017 and 2016. By permission of Scribe Publications on behalf of the Estate of Georgia Blain.

Ciaran Carson: Poems 'Claude Monet, *Artist's Garden at Vétheuil, 1880*'; 'Angela Hackett, *Lemons on a Moorish Plate, 2013*'; 'Canaletto, *The Stonemason's Yard, c. 1725*'; and 'John Constable, *Study of Clouds, 1822*' from *Still Life* (2019). Copyright © Ciaran Carson 2019. Reproduced with kind permission of the Author's Estate and The Gallery Press. www.gallerypress.com

Raymond Carver: Poems 'What the Doctor Said', 'Gravy', 'Through the Boughs' and 'Late Fragment' from *All Of Us*. Published by Harvill Press. Copyright © Raymond Carver 1996. Reprinted by permission of Penguin Books Limited.

J. M. Coetzee: From *Age of Iron*. Published by Secker. Copyright © J.M. Coetzee 1990. Reprinted by permission of Penguin Books Limited.

Mary Costello: Short Story 'Little Disturbances' from *The China Factory*. Published by Canongate Books Ltd. Copyright © Mary Costello 2012. Reproduced with permission of Canongate Books Limited through PLSclear.

Peter De Vries: From *The Blood of the Lamb*. Published by University of Chicago Press, 2005. Copyright © Peter De Vries 1961. By permission of University of Chicago Press.

John Diamond: From *C: Because Cowards Get Cancer Too*. Published by Vermillion. Copyright © John Diamond 1998. Reprinted by permission of Penguin Books Limited.

Helen Dunmore: Poems 'My life's stem was cut' and 'My People' from *Counting Backwards: Poems 1975 – 2017*. Published by Bloodaxe Books. Copyright © Helen Dunmore 2017. Reproduced with permission of Bloodaxe Books. www.bloodaxebooks.com

Elaine Feeney: From *As You Were*. Published by Vintage. Copyright © Elaine Feeney, 2020. Reprinted by permission of Penguin Books Limited.

Neil Gaiman: From 'Why our future depends on libraries, reading and daydreaming'. Copyright © 2013 by Neil Gaiman. Reprinted by permission of Writers House LLC acting as agent for the author.

Helen Garner: From *The Spare Room*. Published by Canongate Books. Copyright © Helen Garner 2008. Reprinted by permission of Canongate Books.

Susan Gubar: From *Reading & Writing Cancer: How Words Heal*. Published by W.W. Norton & Company. Copyright © Susan Gubar, 2016. Reprinted by permission of Susan Gubar.

Donald Hall: Poems 'The Ship Pounding', 'Without' and 'Weeds and Peonies' from *Without: Poems*. Copyright © 1998 by Donald Hall. Used by permission of HarperCollins Publishers.

Philip Hodgins: Poems 'Room 1 Ward 10 West 23/11/83', 'A House in the Country', 'Blood Connections' and 'Wordy Wordy Numb Numb', and excerpts from poems 'Shooting the Dogs', 'Second Thoughts on The Georgics', and 'The Cause of Death'. All from *First Light: a selection of poems*. Published by George Braziller Inc. Copyright © 2015 by Janet Shaw. Reprinted by permission of Janet Shaw, Anna Shaw and Helen Hodgins. All Rights Reserved.

Clive James: Poem 'Elementary Sonnet' from *Sentenced to Life*. Published by Picador, an imprint of Pan Macmillan. Copyright © Clive James 2015. Reproduced with permission of Pan Macmillan through PLSclear.

Jennifer Johnston: Excerpts reproduced from *The Christmas Tree*. Copyright © 1981 by Jennifer Johnston. Reprinted by permission of Jennifer Johnston and the Felix de Wolfe Literary Agency.

EXTENDED COPYRIGHT

Thom Jones: Short Story 'I Want to Live!' from *The Pugilist at Rest*. Copyright © Thom Jones, 1993. Reproduced by permission of Faber & Faber under their fair dealing guidelines.

Clifton Leaf: From *The Truth in Small Doses: Why we're Losing the War on Cancer – and How to Win It*. Copyright © Clifton Leaf. Reprinted with the permission of Simon & Schuster, Inc. All rights reserved.

C.S. Lewis: From *A Grief Observed: Readers' Edition*. Copyright © C.S. Lewis, 1961, 2015. Reproduced by permission of Faber & Faber under their fair dealing guidelines.

Rebecca Loncraine: Reproduced from *Skybound*. Copyright © Estate of Rebecca Loncraine 2018, by permission of United Agents Ltd (www.unitedagents.co.uk) on behalf of the Estate of Rebecca Loncraine.

Audre Lorde: Excerpts from *The Cancer Journals*. Copyright © 1980 by Audre Lorde. Reprinted by permission of Abner Stein Literary Agency. Excerpts from *Burst of Life*. Copyright © 1988 by Audre Lorde. Reprinted by permission of Charlotte Sheedy Literary Agency.

John McGahern: Reproduced from *Memoir*. Copyright © Estate of John McGahern 2005. By permission of Faber and Faber Ltd.

Henning Mankell: From *Quicksand*. Published by Vintage. Copyright © Henning Mankell, 2014. Reprinted by permission of Penguin Books Limited.

Hilary Mantel: From *Giving Up the Ghost: A Memoir*. Copyright © Hilary Mantel, 2003. Published by 4th Estate. Reproduced by permission of A.M. Heath Literary Agents.

Lia Mills: From *In your face: one woman's encounter with cancer, doctors, nurses, machines, family, friends and a few enemies*. Copyright © Lia Mills, 2007. Reprinted by permission of Lia Mills.

Lorrie Moore: Short story 'People Like That Are the Only People Here: Canonical Babbling in Peed Onk' from *Birds of America*. Copyright © Lorrie Moore, 1998. Reproduced by permission of Faber and Faber under their fair dealing guidelines.

Toni Morrison: From Toni Morrison interview, *Cincinnati Enquirer*, 27th September, 1981. Reproduced by permission of Princeton University Library.

Siddhartha Mukherjee: From *The Emperor of All Maladies: A Biography of Cancer*. Published by Fourth Estate. Copyright © Siddhartha Mukherjee, 2011. Reprinted by permissions of HarperCollins Publishers Limited.

THE BREATH OF CONSOLATION

Alice Munro: Short story 'Floating Bridge' from *Hateship, Friendship, Courtship, Loveship, Marriage*. Published by Vintage. Copyright © Alice Munro 2001. Reprinted by permission of Penguin Books Limited.

Patrick Ness: Text © Patrick Ness 2011. From an original idea by Siobhan Dowd. From *A Monster Calls* written by Patrick Ness. Reproduced by permission of Walker Books Ltd, London, SE11 5HJ www.walkerbooks.co.uk

Edna O'Brien: From *Country Girl*. Published by Faber and Faber Copyright © Edna O'Brien, 2012. Reproduced by permission of Edna O'Brien.

Mary Bradish O'Connor: Poems 'Midnight Cancer', 'Venerable Bede in Caspar', 'Say Yes Quickly' and 'Getting Stronger Every Day' from *Say Yes Quickly: A Cancer Tapestry*. Copyright © Pot Shard Press, reprinted with permission from Bored Feet Press LLP.

Tillie Olsen: Short story 'Tell Me a Riddle' from *Tell Me a Riddle & Yonnondio* by Tillie Olsen with introductions by Cora Kaplan. Published by Virago. Copyright © Tillie Olsen 1960, 1961. Reproduced with permission of Little Brown Book Group Limited through PLSclear.

Richard Powers: From *Gain*. Published by William Heinemann. Copyright © Richard Powers, 1998. Reprinted by permission of The Random House Group Limited.

Oliver Sacks: From *Gratitude*. Published by Picador. Copyright © Oliver Sacks 2015. Reproduced with permission of Pan Macmillan through PLSclear.

Bernhard Schlink: Short story 'The Last Summer' from *Summer Lies,* translated by Carol Brown Janeway. Published by Weidenfeld & Nicolson. Copyright © Bernhard Schlink and Carol Brown Janeway, 2010, 2012. Reproduced with permission of Orion Publishing Group Limited through PLSclear.

Jo Shapcott: Poems 'Of Mutability', 'Hairless', 'Stargazer' and 'Procedure' from *Of Mutability* by Jo Shapcott published by Faber and Faber limited. Copyright © Jo Shapcott, 2010. Reproduced by permission of Faber and Faber Limited.

Lionel Shriver: From *So Much For That*. Published by HarperCollins Publishers Ltd. Copyright © Lionel Shriver, 2010. Reprinted by permission of HarperCollins Publishers Ltd.

Rebecca Skloot: From *The Immortal Life of Henrietta Lacks*. Published by Macmillan, an imprint of Pan Macmillan. Copyright © Rebecca Skloot, 2010. Reproduced by permission of Macmillan Publishers International Limited.

EXTENDED COPYRIGHT

Marin Sorescu: Poems 'The Bridge' and 'The Cowardly Coffin' from *The Bridge*. Translated by Adam J. Sorkin and Lidia Vianu. Published by Bloodaxe Books (2004). Copyright © Marin Sorescu, Adam Sorkin and Lidia Vianu. Reproduced with permission of Bloodaxe Books. www.bloodaxebooks.com

Elizabeth Strout: Short story 'Light' from *Olive, Again*. Published by Penguin. Copyright © Elizabeth Strout 2019. Reprinted by permission of Penguin Books Limited.

Colm Toibín: From *A Guest at the Feast*. Published by Viking. Copyright © Colm Tóibín, 2022. Reprinted by permission of Penguin Books Limited.

Leo Tolstoy: From *The Death of Ivan Ilych And Confession*. Translated by Peter Carson. Copyright © 2014 by The Estate of Peter Carson. Used by permission of Liveright Publishing Corporation.

Alberto Barrera Tyszka: From *The Sickness*. Translated by Margaret Jull Costa. Published by Quercus Publishing Limited. Copyright © Alberto Barrera Tyszka and Margaret Jull Costa 2010. Reproduced with permission of Quercus Publishing Limited through PLSclear.

Althea H. Warren: From her speech 'Read Without Weeping' given at the Twenty-Sixth Annual Conference of the Pacific Northwest Library Association, 1935, Portland, Oregon. Reproduced with no objections from Simon & Schuster or from the American Library Association.

Christian Wiman: Excerpts from *My Bright Abyss*. Copyright © 2013 by Christian Wiman. Reprinted by permission of Farrar, Straus and Giroux. All Rights Reserved. Poems 'After the Diagnosis', 'This Mind of Dying', 'Every Riven Thing' and 'Gone for The Day, She is the Day' from *Every Riven Thing*. Copyright © 2010 by Christian Wiman. Reprinted by permission of Farrar, Straus and Giroux. All Rights Reserved.

Every effort has been made to trace copyright holders and to obtain their permission for the use of copyright material. The author apologises for any errors or omissions in the above list.